Methods in Speech and Language Pathology Series

Methods in Clinical Phonetics

Methods in Clinical Phonetics

MARTIN J. BALL PhD
University of Louisiana at Lafayette

and

ORLA M. LOWRY PhD
University of Ulster

W

WHURR PUBLISHERS
LONDON AND PHILADELPHIA

© 2001 Whurr Publishers
First published 2001 by
Whurr Publishers Ltd
19B Compton Terrace, London N1 2UN, England and
325 Chestnut Street, Philadelphia PA 19106, USA

British Library Cataloguing in Publication Data
A catalogue record for this book is available from the
British Library.

ISBN: 1 86156 184 9

Printed and bound in the UK by Athenaeum Press Ltd,
Gateshead, Tyne & Wear

Contents

Series Preface   **ix**
Introduction   **xi**

Chapter 1   1

What is Clinical Phonetics?

Chapter 2   10

Transcribing Phonetic Data

Chapter 3   25

Transcribing Disordered Speech

Chapter 4   41

Articulatory Instrumentation

Chapter 5   49

Articulatory Analysis of Disordered Speech

Chapter 6   61

Acoustic Instrumentation

Chapter 7   73

Acoustic Analysis of Disordered Speech

Chapter 8   88

Auditory and Perceptual Instrumentation

Chapter 9   99

Auditory and Perceptual Analysis of Disordered Speech

Chapter 10   110

The Future of Clinical Phonetics

References   121
Appendix
   The International Phonetic Alphabet   127
   The Extensions to the International Phonetic Alphabet   128
   The VoQS Voice Quality Symbols   129

Index   131

For
Chris Code

'Ka ia akoakomaiagia ki matou: lea lahi ke ko lagona'

Series Preface

The aim of this series is to provide accessible and relevant texts to students of speech and language disorders and to speech-language pathologists and therapists. The volumes aim to cover a wide variety of topics relevant to such an audience, and to introduce these topics in a practical way to enable student practitioners and qualified clinicians to undertake a range of analysis and treatment procedures. A minimum of background knowledge is assumed for each text, but the books also point readers in the direction of further, more advanced, research.

We intend to cover aspects of clinical linguistics and phonetics as applied to the assessment of speech and language disorders, and aspects of therapeutics suitable for the treatment of the wide range of communication disorders encountered in the clinic. Each volume will be written by leading authorities in the field who have a grasp of both the theoretical issues and the practical requirements of the area and, further, are at the forefront of current research and practice.

This series, then, will act as a bridge between scientific developments in the study of speech and language disorders, and the application of these to clinical assessment and intervention. It is hoped that the texts will stimulate the reader's interest in the topic as well as providing hands-on advice. In this way we can promote well-informed and competent clinicians.

Martin J. Ball, University of Louisiana at Lafayette, USA
Thomas W. Powell, Louisiana State University, USA
and Alison Ferguson, University of Newcastle, NSW, Australia

Introduction

This book introduces the reader to a range of methods in the clinical application of phonetics. Phonetics – the science of speech production, transmission and reception – has long been a vital part of the training of speech-language pathologists and therapists. However, in recent years there has been a remarkable increase in the range of phonetic instrumentation, and notable developments in the area of phonetic transcription. Many of these new techniques have been especially designed for clinical phoneticians, or are equally useful for the clinical and non-clinical researcher. It is the purpose of this book to describe many of these developments, and to guide the reader in how to use them.

The book opens with an account of what clinical phonetics actually is. We argue that phonetics should be considered one of the sciences, and go on to explore its application to speech production (with its links to anatomy and physiology, and aerodynamics), speech transmission (linked to acoustics), and speech reception (connected to audiology). This chapter also describes a range of speech disorders and their phonetic consequences.

The next eight chapters are grouped in pairs: one chapter dealing with theoretical phonetic issues, and the following one demonstrating the application of this area to disordered speech. Chapter 2 deals with impressionistic transcription, describing the International Phonetic Alphabet and how it is used. Chapter 3 introduces recent additions to the transcriber's armoury to help in the transcription of speech disorders, and of voice quality (both normal and disordered). Throughout these chapters, the importance of narrow transcription is stressed, and examples are given of the problems that arise if transcriptions are restricted to the phonemic level of the target language.

Chapter 4 deals with instrumentation designed to help analyse speech articulation. This ranges from electromyography – designed to examine the electrical activity in speech muscles – through electrolaryngography/

electroglottography (which looks at vocal fold activity), to electropalatography (measuring tongue–palate contact in real time during speech),
among others. Of course, some of these techniques are more useful to the
clinical phonetician than others (especially if they have a therapeutic
application as well as a purely research one), and these are explored in
Chapter 5. This chapter describes a series of studies using electropalatography, electrolaryngography and nasometry.

In Chapter 6 we look at how phoneticians undertake acoustic analysis.
This involves the use of sound spectrography, made much more accessible
recently through developments in software for personal computers. A
range of measures applied to various types of speech sound are described
and illustrated. In Chapter 7 we look at how sound spectrography can
help us describe disfluent speech, unusual vowel qualities, and segment
durations in dysarthric speech.

Chapter 8 describes the two major methodologies in auditory
phonetics: delayed auditory feedback and dichotic listening. In Chapter 9
we describe some important studies that have used these techniques in
the investigation of aphasia and disfluency. Our final chapter presents a
brief look at possible future developments in clinical phonetics. We are
beginning to see the integration of different measures (e.g. spectrographic
and articulatory) in modern instruments, and the greater use of PC-based
packages. It is also possible that some of the imaging techniques (such as
electromagnetic articulography) may become smaller, cheaper and easier
to use. It is an exciting time to work in clinical phonetics!

CHAPTER 1
What is Clinical Phonetics?

In this book, we are concerned with methods in clinical phonetics, but before we can start on this task we need to be clear what the field of clinical phonetics actually is. We shall start by looking at the science of phonetics itself, and situate clinical phonetics in relation to its broader discipline.

Phonetics is normally defined as being the 'scientific study of speech sounds'. The different aspects of this definition can be examined in turn. First, we shall consider what constitutes the subject material of phonetics: speech sounds. It should be noted that speech sounds include all aspects of sound used in speech, and this includes vowel sounds, consonant sounds, and aspects of speech such as intonation and rhythm, loudness and tempo. There are some sounds produced by speakers that are peripheral to this definition. For example, we can produce a range of sounds that are generally considered to be extralinguistic – that is to say they do not fit into the linguistic systems of consonants, vowels, etc. These include hestitation noises, annoyance or encouragement clicks (e.g. as written 'tut-tut'), sighs, and so on. Although it is clear that these sounds do not operate in the same way as the main linguistic sound units referred to above, they often do have some kind of meaning attached to them, and linguists studying the mechanics of conversation usually include these sound types in their analyses. It should be stressed here, however, that sounds that are extralinguistic in one language may well constitute part of the consonant system of others. For example, we mentioned above the annoyance and encouragement clicks; although these do not play a linguistic role in English, they are treated as part of the consonant systems of a range of (mainly) southern African languages. This stresses the need to include within the body of speech sounds that are studied in phonetics, all sounds used linguistically in natural language – whatever the language.

1

The other aspect of our original definition was 'scientific study'. By this we mean that phoneticians attempt a comprehensive, systematic, and objective account of the speech data they are describing. These descriptions may be based on the auditory impressions of the phoneticians, but these impressions will normally be translated into an internationally agreed system of symbolization and/or articulatory labels, in which the phonetician has been rigorously trained. However, increasingly frequently, phoneticians are using a range of instrumentation to investigate the articulatory, acoustic and perceptual aspects of speech. Although these instrumental techniques still contain a degree of uncertainty (in that interpreting read-outs from many pieces of equipment is not always straightforward), they do eliminate a considerable amount of unavoidable subjective influence on the interpretation of data that must impinge on impressionistic transcription of speech.

Modern phonetics, then, is partly interested in providing descriptions of speech data using as scientific an approach as possible. The move towards a greater use of instrumental techniques does not mean, however, that traditional impressionistic transcription using phonetic symbols is about to be abandoned. There are many instances when phoneticians do not have immediate or easy access to instrumentation, and indeed, when reading off results from many types of phonetic equipment, it is often easiest to state these in terms of phonetic symbols. In recent times, we have begun to see a marrying together of the two approaches, with instrumental evidence being used to help to solve transcription problems (see Ball and Rahilly 1996).

Nevertheless, phonetics is also interested in theory building, on the basis of descriptions of speech behaviours that have been provided over the years. In other words, our knowledge of speech behaviour gained from both impressionistic and instrumental analysis can inform our ideas on the complex speech chain from speech production through to speech perception. In investigating theories of speech production and perception we shall be accessing interdisciplinary areas such as neurolinguistics and neurophonetics in the study of speech production, and psychoacoustics in the study of speech perception.

We also need to bear in mind that phonetics is concerned with all aspects of speech: that is to say, not just the production of speech sounds by a speaker, but their transmission through air, and their perception by the hearer. These aspects of spoken communication are often given separate labels in phonetics (see Ball 1993):

* *articulatory phonetics* (the use of the vocal organs to produce sounds)
* *acoustic phonetics* (the study of the sound waves of speech)

- *auditory phonetics* (the study of the reception of speech sounds by the hearer).

These terms are, however, somewhat too limited. For example, in investigating the reception of speech sounds we may not be interested only in the physical activity of the auditory system, but also in the way in which the brain sorts out and interprets the incoming signals decoded by that system; in other words, how we perceive speech. Therefore, perceptual phonetics has come to be examined in its own right, as the step beyond the purely physical auditory process.

Also, articulatory phonetics can be viewed as not the first step in the procedure of creating a spoken message. Preceding articulatory activity, there must be activity in the brain to organize and plan an utterance. Higher-level linguistic aspects of this planning (e.g. the semantics, syntax and phonology of a message) are beyond the scope of phonetics, of course. Nevertheless, it is clear that phonetic plans must be created and implemented neurologically in order for a spoken message to be initiated. Neurophonetics is a term that can be applied to this area of study (as noted earlier), and is an important area within clinical phonetics as it can be subject to disruption in some types of disorder.

We have only scratched the surface here of what phonetics is about, and readers new to the topic are recommended to consult one of a number of excellent texts in phonetics that have been published in the last few years: Ball (1993), Clark and Yallop (1995), Ladefoged (1993), Laver (1994), Ball and Rahilly (1999).

Clinical phonetics

If phonetics is the scientific study and description of speech sounds, then clinical phonetics is the application of this approach to the speech sounds used by speakers with a speech problem. Of course, there is a wide range of speech problems, and each has its own effect on a speaker's abilities. We shall, therefore, look in turn at the most commonly occurring speech disorders, and consider what their clinical phonetic characteristics are.

We shall start this brief survey by considering types of disorder that have a physical origin (in most instances), and affect the speaker's ability to produce sounds. The first of these that we shall consider is commonly known as 'cleft palate', though a more usual term these days is *craniofacial disorders*, as this covers a set of related problems that do not consist solely of clefts in the palate. Incomplete formation of the palate, and other disorders that affect the ability to close off the nasal cavity from the oral cavity during speech (*velopharyngeal inadequacy*), have perhaps the greatest impact on the intelligibility of speech of all the craniofacial disorders. First, as we have just noted, this type of problem will create a difficulty in maintaining a contrast between oral and nasal sounds. This means that vowels and sonorants (e.g. central and lateral approximants) are likely to be pronounced with excessive nasality,[1] and plosive stops may be replaced by nasal stops.

Another problem that cleft palate speakers have is to maintain intra-oral air pressure, as the cleft allows air to escape into the nasal cavity. Such pressure is important in the production of plosives of course, but also of fricatives, as a turbulent airflow, necessary for such sounds, is difficult to maintain without adequate intra-oral air pressure. In less severe cases, nasalized stops (i.e. not fully nasal stops, but oral stops with concomitant nasal air release and weak plosion) and nasalized fricatives occur; in more severe cases, plosives may be realized as fully nasal stops, and fricatives as nasal stops with accompanying nasal friction (that is to say turbulent airflow through the nasal cavity), these being voiceless in the case of voiceless fricative targets. This combination of features tends to make cleft palate speech difficult to understand (and also difficult to transcribe phonetically; we return to this point in Chapter 3).

We can also consider voice disorders under a general heading of disorders with a physical origin. Although it is possible that some voice disorders do not have purely physical origins, most of them can be traced to some problem with the vocal folds or associated laryngeal structures or the neurological control of these structures. We do not have the space here to go into this large area of study in any detail, but we can point to some of the phonetic consequences of vocal disorder. The activity of the vocal folds and larynx as a whole in speech is important in several ways. The major distinction of phonation types between voiced and voiceless consonants is found in all natural language. Voice disorders that inhibit the consistent production of this distinction will obviously impact heavily on a speaker's intelligibility.

Further, pitch differences in speech (used for example in the intonation system of a language) depend on laryngeal activity; therefore, a voice disorder could also affect the ability to control intonation patterns. Although intonation may appear secondary to the production of segmental aspects of speech (i.e. consonants and vowels), impaired intonation can often cause communicative breakdown through listeners misunderstanding the communicative intent of a speaker (e.g. thinking that a comment is intended as an order).

---

[1] It should be recognized that to some extent nasality in such contexts may differ in normal speakers in terms of regional accent. However, the hypernasality found with cleft palate speakers, combined with other features of their speech, is rarely confusable with normal nasality in these accents.

Voice disorders may not affect (or not only affect) these linguistic systems. They may change the overall voice quality of a speaker to one that has a highly breathy quality, or one where creak predominates, or a harsh quality perhaps through utilizing the ventricular folds as well as, or instead of, the vocal folds. Although these changes may not impair the ability to signal voiced–voiceless distinctions, they can be very distressing to the speaker. All these suprasegmental aspects of speech will need to be described as accurately as possible by the clinical phonetician, and in some of these areas there are not always widely accepted means of transcribing them. We return to this difficulty in Chapter 3.

Another group of disorders can be grouped together under a general heading of *child speech disorders*. There are various competing attempts to subdivide these. Some researchers have classified them in terms of whether the disorder primarily affects phonological organization or phonetic realization; others have adopted a strategy of dividing disordered child speech into one type exhibiting signs of delayed normal development, and another showing deviant patterns. Recent research suggests that both of these approaches are too simplistic, and what is needed is a typology that takes both these aspects into consideration. Following work by Dodd and her colleagues (see, for example, Dodd 1995, Holm and Dodd 1999), we suggest here that four main types of child speech disorder can be recognized: delayed normal, consistent deviant, inconsistent deviant and developmental verbal dyspraxia (DVD). We do not have space here to go into the debate concerning this classification (particularly of the much debated DVD category), but readers interested in this area should see the Further Reading section below.

Although the delayed normal group of child speech disorders generally exhibits patterns of phonological simplifications that can be transcribed straightforwardly by clinical phoneticians capable of transcribing the target system phonemically (but even here some phonetic differences may need to be recorded), the other three groups may exhibit a wide range of speech patterns including some very atypical ones. These may well include sounds not found in natural language, as well as sounds from outside the target phonological system. The phonetician, therefore, may need to describe sounds using places and manners of articulation not listed for normal speech. It is clear, then, that in these instances clinical phonetics must stretch both the terminology and the symbolization provided by phonetic theory.

The next area we can examine includes disorders that fall under the heading of dysfluency. The two main types of fluency disorder are stuttering and cluttering, though the bulk of research into fluency is concerned with the former. Disfluent speakers may exhibit a wide range of behaviours apart from repetitions of segments or of groups of segments. However, even repetitions present difficulties in terms of phonetic description. Without recourse to acoustic instrumentation it may well be very difficult to count accurately the number of repetitions that take place as they may be very rapid, or very quiet. On the purely transcriptional level, there has until recently been no agreed way of transcribing a stuttered repetition, or of showing pauses that often accompany stuttering episodes.

Other features of speech that commonly occur with more severe stutterers include changes in voice quality (breathy and creaky can occur), extra strong articulations following a block, use of ingressive airflow, and atypical sounds such as the velopharyngeal fricative or 'snort'. With clutterers, one feature that is common is excessively fast tempo, while stutterers may also demonstrate changes in tempo and in loudness. Many of these features are suprasegmental aspects of speech, and it is often the case that these aspects are not dealt with as thoroughly as segmental ones in phonetics courses. Clinical phoneticians must, therefore, be aware of suprasegmentals and be equipped to describe them both instrumentally and through transcription. We return to both these techniques in later chapters in the book.

The next group of disorders we shall consider are those acquired after head injury or stroke, often termed *acquired neurological disorders*. One of the main areas of interest in this group is *aphasia*, or acquired language disorder. There are several sub-types of aphasia (and numerous competing classifications and labels), and it is not part of the scope of this book to go into these in detail. What we need to bear in mind, however, is a basic distinction between receptive (or Wernicke's type) aphasia, and productive (or Broca's type). Clearly, it is the productive type or types that will be of most interest to the clinical phonetician, and, of course, the phonological aspects (as opposed to semantic, syntactic, pragmatic, etc. aspects). Among these phonological aspects we may find dysprosody, specifically inappropriate use of intonation; frequent use of filled and unfilled pauses; phonological paraphasias (such as substitutions, transpositions and additions of sounds); and repetitions and perseverations.

Aphasic clients also often display a wide range of receptive and expressive linguistic difficulties other than phonological ones. These may involve the lexicon (word-finding difficulties, semantic paraphasias), syntax, semantics and pragmatics. It is not always easy to allocate a particular linguistic behaviour to any of these categories, however. Repetitions of segments or syllables, hesitations and perseverations may all be a result of a problem at another level (such as word-finding difficulty). It must be stressed, therefore, that aphasic speakers must be assessed in as broad a way as possible. Nevertheless, it is important that an accurate description of their speech behaviours is available to be part of an overall description of their language problems.

Speakers with aphasia may also suffer from one of the other two phonetically important acquired neurological disorders – *apraxia of speech* and *dysarthria* – or these disorders can also occur without aphasia.[2] Apraxia of speech is a disorder of motor programming; in other words, the speaker cannot put into effect what they have planned to say (as opposed to aphasia where the correct motor plans cannot even be drawn up). The disorder in apraxia is not due to problems with the nervous system or the muscles of speech, it is with the volitional control over the system. Apraxic speakers can often produce utterances casually (such as a greeting or other common saying), but when asked to produce the utterance on another occasion will be unable to do so.

A wide range of phonetic and phonological problems may be evidenced, depending on the subject. For example, the use of voice with obstruent consonants (i.e. stops, fricatives and affricates) may be impossible, although voice is used perfectly normally with sonorant consonants and vowels.[3] To compensate for this problem, a patient reported in Code and Ball (1982) made use of the fact that vowels in front of voiced obstruents are longer than the same vowels in front of voiceless ones. This patient maintained the vowel length differences (and incidentally lengthened the amount of frication considerably more than usual) as a means of signalling the contrast between voiced and voiceless fricatives, as the normal voicing aspect was impossible to use.

Dysarthria differs from apraxia of speech in that the impairment is one of motor execution rather than planning. Various types of damage to different parts of the neuromuscular system responsible for speech will result in dysarthria (we shall not go into the sub-types of the disorder here). Depending on the location of the damage, various phonetic consequences will be manifested: problems of airstream initiation, phonation, segmental articulation or suprasegmental control.

For example, a patient described in Ball *et al* (1994) was described as having a spastic dysarthria characterized predominately by a harsh, strained-strangled voice, and monopitch, monoloudness and nasal emission. Articulation was severely impaired and characterized by imprecise consonant production. Although the patient could achieve restricted lip movement, tongue elevation was very restricted anteriorly and posteriorly. A transcription of this patient's speech is found in the article cited.

---

[2] Both these disorders can be developmental as well as acquired.

[3] This is good evidence to support the idea that voiced obstruents are less natural than voiceless ones, but that the reverse is true for sonorants

Hearing impairment may not seem to be an obvious category in our survey of speech disorders. However, the removal of the auditory feedback route does cause some fairly consistent problems with speech production. That this does occur supports the belief of phoneticians that feedback is an important part of monitoring our accuracy in speaking, and that specific feedback routes (auditory being one of these) help control specific aspects of speech. However, before we look at the phonetics of the hearing impaired in any more detail, we must bear in mind that two main categories of these speakers exist: the prelingually deaf, and the postlingually deafened. With the first of these categories, the fact that hearing was lost before language developed (or was absent from birth) means that these speakers have never had access to auditory feedback to help them establish accurate speech patterns (though other feedback mechanisms may compensate to some degree here, providing guidance is forthcoming). The postlingual group of speakers have lost their auditory feedback system to a greater or lesser extent after acquiring normal language. With this group, therefore, we witness the gradual erosion over time of accuracy in speech, but alternative feedback routes in therapy (such as vision) may help overcome some of this erosion.

With both groups we may see problems with the articulation of vowels and consonants, and with suprasegmentals. With vowels a variety of patterns are found depending on whether the speaker is pre- or postlingually impaired. In the latter group, for example, there is a tendency for non-fully closed vowels to become more close, and non-fully open vowels to become more open, along with competing patterns of monophthongization and diphthongization. For consonants there is a tendency for labial consonants to be more accurately preserved than non-labials (especially with prelingually deaf speakers who use lip-reading). Indeed, many non-labials may be subject to deletion or replacement by glottal stop. Among many other reported problems are difficulties with fricatives and the simplification of clusters.

Disruption to suprasegmental aspects of speech is often thought of as a major problem with hearing-impaired speakers, and it is clear that the auditory feedback route is used by non-hearing-impaired speakers primarily to control such aspects. This disruption may manifest itself in problems with loudness and tempo, stress and intonation, though, unfortunately, the reports show little consistency as to the direction the changes take.

It is clear from this brief survey of hearing-impaired speech that clinical phoneticians must be equipped to describe a wide range of both segmental and suprasegmental disorders. As problems with intonation figure largely in reports of these clients, we must be able to analyse this aspect of the speech signal in a coherent and consistent manner.

Conclusion

This chapter has presented only a brief survey of disorders that can have possible implications for speech production, and does not claim to be comprehensive (for example, we have not touched on areas such as cognitive disorders, including autism and learning difficulties). We have not looked in detail at (non-phonological) linguistic disorders, or disorders of reception of language, though there may well be overlaps between these and speech production disorders. We have also not distinguished between disorders that have traditionally been termed phonetic and those termed phonological. The reason for this is that it is often difficult to tell the difference, and in any case detailed clinical phonetic description of all speech disorders is needed before we can tell at what level of organization the disorder is operating: earlier clear-cut distinctions no longer seem so reliable (see Kent 1996). It is the aim of this book to show you how you can undertake these descriptions, and so aid your remediation planning and execution.

Further reading

This book is not an introduction to phonetic theory, but readers will have to know the basics of phonetics to understand much of the discussion in this and other chapters. They are recommended, therefore, to consult such books as Ball (1993), Ball and Rahilly (1999), Catford (1988), Clark and Yallop (1995), Ladefoged (1993) and Laver (1994).

Neither is it an introduction to speech and language pathology, for which an introductory text such as Crystal and Varley (1998) would serve well. Such a work will provide further references for research into specific disorders, and we shall not provide a full list of these here. We can mention, however, work by Dodd (1995), Bradford and Dodd (1996) and Holm and Dodd (1999) on the classification of child speech disorders. We also noted above that dysarthria was not described in any detail, and readers should consult Darley, Aronson and Brown (1975) for further information. Kent (1996) provides a good overview of developments in theoretical issues.

CHAPTER 2

Transcribing Phonetic Data

When we describe speech we can take either an impressionistic approach or an instrumental one (or, as we shall see later, a combination of both of these). Instrumental approaches to the description of speech are described in detail in later chapters of this book; here, we concentrate on the impressionistic method.

Impressionistic description is normally realized through the use of phonetic transcription. In transcription we use a set of graphic symbols on paper to stand for aspects of the speech signal: it is impressionistic because we can write down only those aspects that we can perceive, in other words we record our impressions of the signal. There have been numerous attempts in the history of phonetics to devise adequate symbol systems for recording impressionistic transcriptions (see Abercrombie 1967, Ball, Rahilly and Tench 1996), but the generally accepted standard system today is the *International Phonetic Alphabet* (IPA), and this is the system used in this book. Some scholars, particularly in North America, and those working with theoretical phonology,[1] use a slightly different system often termed the *Americanist tradition*.[2] Most of these differences are relatively slight, affecting a small number of symbols. We shall point these differences out in relevant places later in this chapter when we look at the specific symbols we need to transcribe speech.

---

[1] Phonologists construct rigorous theories to account for the patterns of sounds used in specific languages and across languages as a whole. Phonology can also be used clinically to examine patterns of disordered speech and revise remediation strategies. This area is outside the scope of this book, but will be covered in a later volume in the series.

[2] Under this broad heading we can include the slight changes in basic symbols, such as [y] for IPA [j], but also the diacritics and other symbols of the Summer Institute of Linguistics which also differ from IPA norms.

What do we transcribe?

We have so far talked about transcribing the speech signal graphically via a symbol set such as the IPA. However, we have also to ask what aspects of the speech signal we transcribe. As suggested above, certain aspects of the acoustic signal are difficult or impossible to transcribe impressionistically as we cannot hear them or cannot hear them very accurately (such as minute differences in the length in time of aspects of a sound). But beyond those aspects, we still have to decide which features of spoken language we wish to record. Most obvious, perhaps, are the so-called *segments*[3] of speech: the consonants and the vowels.

A word of caution is needed here. The terms 'consonant' and 'vowel' are used in everyday parlance to refer to the letters of the alphabet used in the ordinary orthography (i.e. writing system) of English, or any other language using an alphabetic approach to writing.[4] However, in English the number of consonant letters or vowel letters may bear little resemblance to the number of consonant sounds or vowel sounds, owing to the lack of a direct equivalence between sound and symbol. For example, 'rough' has only three sounds (a consonant at the beginning, a vowel in the middle and a consonant at the end: speak it out loud to test it), but it has five letters, three of them consonant letters and two of them vowel letters. We return to the problem of written English in more detail below.

Apart from the consonants and vowels, however, there are many other aspects of speech that may need to be recorded (especially if we are looking at speakers with speech disorders). These non-segmental features are often termed 'suprasegmental' or 'prosodic' aspects of speech. They cover the rhythmic characteristics of a spoken utterance (e.g. in terms of the placement of stressed and unstressed syllables); intonation (the placement of pitch movements across an utterance); voice quality (the use of breathy or creaky voice, for example); tempo (the speed and changes in speed used by the speaker); and loudness. Some or all of these features may be important to a total understanding of the message, or to the complete characterization of a speaker's abilities, and so we must have more than an *ad hoc* way of recording them.

---

[3] We shall see later that speech cannot be divided into neat segments as easily as is traditionally thought.

[4] Such as the Latin alphabet we use, the Cyrillic alphabet of Russian and the Greek alphabet. Other systems are based on syllables or parts of words, and for these terms like consonant and vowel will be irrelevant as applied to writing.

We might also be interested in the way speakers manage discourse, or conversation, between each other. In this respect, we may wish to be able to record features that occur in conversations, such as pauses, hesitation noises, overlapping speech between two speakers, and so on. However, whatever aspects of speech we decide to transcribe, we must have a widely-known and respected system to transcribe with.

What do we transcribe with?

It might be thought that we can undertake a phonetic transcription simply by using the ordinary writing system that we currently use when writing English. However, as we saw above, the number of consonants and vowels in terms of written letters does not always correspond directly to the number of spoken vowels and consonants.

We are also plagued with the problem that in English the same sound can be represented by different spellings. The 'f' sound can be spelt in any of the following ways:

f	if
ff	off
gh	cough
ph	graph

With vowels it can be even worse. The 'ee' sound of English can be spelt in any of the following ways:

ee	see
ea	sea
ei	deceive
ie	piece
y	beauty
i	police
e	me

Unfortunately, the converse problem also arises. The same spelling can be used to represent several different pronunciations. Let's look at a couple of examples:

'ng'	as in	singer	(no 'g' pronounced)
		finger	('g' pronounced)
		whinger	('g' pronounced as 'j')

Again, we find it is often more common with vowels:

'ow'	as in 'cow' or as in 'low'
'ie'	as in 'piece' or as in 'lie'
'i'	as in 'hit' or as in 'police' or as in 'like'

We could have listed many more examples, but the conclusion we must come to is that English orthography presents two important problems to any phonetician wanting to make an accurate record of spoken language: a symbol does not always represent the same pronunciation, and a pronunciation can be represented by a range of different symbols. There is also another problem we must face. As English has more consonant and vowel sounds (particularly vowels) than we have consonant and vowel letters, we are forced to use double combinations of letters to represent single sounds. The following are all common examples:[5]

'th', 'sh', 'ch', 'ee', 'oo'

The problem with this approach is that people may come to feel that sounds represented this way are somehow double sounds, and expect that the beginning of the word 'ship', for example, is made up of an 's' sound followed by an 'h' sound. Try saying that combination, and you'll soon find it doesn't make a 'sh'! We need to ensure, therefore, that a phonetic symbol system uses only one symbol when a single sound is being transcribed.

We can also note that sometimes we find a symbol that can stand for a cluster of two sounds. 'X' in words like 'extra' or 'example' represents a 'k' sound followed by an 's' sound (or for some speakers in some of these words, a 'g' sound followed by a 'z' sound). There is also the problem that at the beginning of words 'x' is basically another way of writing 'z' ('xylophone'). It is clearly a waste of a good symbol in this instance, and we would want to avoid having a single symbol to stand for a combination that can quite easily be represented by two separate symbols.

We can recapitulate, then, what we should need in an adequate phonetic transcription system.

---

[5] Some of these examples also demonstrate the problem that spellings can represent different pronunciations. 'Th' can represent two different pronunciations: compare the sound in 'thin' with the sound in 'then'. Likewise, 'oo' can stand for the long vowel in 'boot' and the short vowel in 'book' for most English accents.

- First, we must ensure that every symbol used in the system represents only one pronunciation, so that when we see a symbol we now precisely how to pronounce it.
- Second, we need to make sure that every pronunciation is represented by only one symbolization, so that when we hear a sound we know precisely how to write it down in transcription. We want to avoid double symbols or any combination of symbols representing single sounds, and we want to avoid single symbols representing double sounds.

The system that comes closest to meeting these goals is normally recognized to be the International Phonetic Alphabet (IPA), and we look at that system in the next section.

The International Phonetic Alphabet

The IPA was first drawn up in 1888 (Ball, Rahilly and Tench 1996 give a more detailed history of the development of this alphabet), but has been subject to numerous additions and amendments since then. The most recent changes date from 1989, with the chart that sets out the symbols appearing in its current shape in 1993 (and slightly amended in 1996). The alphabet is regulated by the International Phonetic Association (also known as IPA: this ambiguity between the abbreviation for the association and for the alphabet is deliberate), and we show the current version of the IPA chart in the Appendix at the end of the book. We also reproduce sections of the chart in this chapter.

If we examine the chart, we can see that it consists of several sections, and we shall examine these in turn. At the top left of the chart is the consonants section (Figure 2.1) (which in turn consists of a chart containing a series of rows and columns, at the intersections of which

	Bilabial	Labiodental	Dental	Alveolar	Postalveolar	Retroflex	Palatal	Velar	Uvular	Pharyngeal	Glottal
Plosive	p b			t d		ʈ ɖ	c ɟ	k g	q ɢ		ʔ
Nasal	m	ɱ		n		ɳ	ɲ	ŋ	N		
Trill	ʙ			r					R		
Tap or Flap				ɾ		ɽ					
Fricative	ɸ β	f v	θ ð	s z	ʃ ʒ	ʂ ʐ	ç ʝ	x ɣ	χ ʁ	ħ ʕ	h ɦ
Lateral fricative				ɬ ɮ							
Approximant		ʋ		ɹ		ɻ	j	ɰ			
Lateral approximant				l		ɭ	ʎ	ʟ			

Figure 2.1. Pulmonic consonant section of the IPA chart (revised to 1993, corrected 1996). Where symbols appear in pairs, the one to the right represents a voiced consonant. Shaded areas denote articulations judged impossible.

are boxes, many of which contain phonetic symbols). The first thing we notice is that many of these symbols are familiar to us, as they appear identical to many of the letters we use to write English. However, although this can often be a help in learning the phonetic symbols, we must remember two things. First, some of the symbols may have different values to those that we associate with the orthographic letter (e.g. [x] and [q]),[6] and second the IPA symbols are used in a consistent manner (e.g. [g] always represents the 'hard' sound in 'get', never the 'soft' sound in 'gin').

The consonant chart contains a large number of symbols, and not all these are needed to transcribe English phonetically. As this is the *International* Phonetic Alphabet, it must obviously contain symbols for the sounds of as many languages as possible, so there will be many symbols we do not need for English. Nevertheless, it is important that students of phonetics learn to make and recognize as many sound distinctions as possible, particularly when dealing with speech dis-ordered clients, as they may well produce a range of non-English sounds.

The chart also contains some empty boxes. Those empty boxes that are shaded on the chart represent articulations that it is deemed impossible to make; unshaded empty boxes are possible sounds for which no symbol is provided. This may be because the sounds are very rare in natural language, or indeed have never been reported in natural language. Some of these articulations may be found in atypical speech as encountered clinically, so there is an extra chart for symbols for such sounds, which we shall examine in Chapter 3.

The consonant chart is in fact three-dimensional:

- the rows represent manners of articulation: plosive stop, nasal stop, fricative, etc.
- the columns represent places of articulation: bilabial, labio-dental, alveolar, velar, etc.
- within each box the left-hand symbol represents the voiceless con-sonant and the right-hand symbol stands for the voiced equivalent.[7]

Some boxes contain only a voiced symbol (e.g. [j] and [l]). In these cases, voiceless equivalents are rare in natural language, and when they do occur they can be transcribed with the voiced symbol plus an extra diacritic (like

---

[6] From now on, we shall put phonetic symbols in square brackets, as is the accepted norm, to distinguish them from orthographic letters.
[7] For descriptions of the terms used here for place and manner of articulation and voicing, see any of the recommended texts on phonetic theory, such as Ball (1993).

an accent mark) which stands for voiceless; we shall look at diacritics later. One exception to this is the symbol for the glottal stop ([ʔ]): as this sound is formed by closing the vocal folds completely, it is neither voiced nor voiceless. On the chart, it is placed on the left in its box, and the right-hand side is shaded to show that a voiced glottal stop is impossible. In this instance, the left-hand side has to be interpreted as non-voiced, rather than as voiceless with open glottis.

From this consonant chart, we need the following symbols to transcribe most accents of English: the plosives [p, t, k, b, d, g] (note that [c] is not used to transcribe the sounds in 'cat' and 'mac'); from the nasals [m, n, ŋ] (this last is used for the 'ng' in 'singer'); from the fricatives we need [f, v, θ, ð, s, z, ʃ, ʒ, h] ([θ] is the 'th' in 'thin', whereas [ð] is the 'th' in 'then', [ʃ] is the 'sh' in 'shop', and [ʒ] is the 's' in 'treasure'); the approximants [ɹ, j] together with [w] from the 'other symbols' part of the overall chart.[8] (English 'r' sounds are often transcribed [r] for ease of recognition, though the approximant quality of 'r' in most English accents should properly have the [ɹ] symbol; [j] is the IPA symbol for 'y' in 'yes': don't use it for the 'j' in 'jam'!)[9] Finally, we need the [l] symbol from the lateral approximant part of the consonant chart to transcribe English 'l'.

Beneath the consonants chart at the left we have the non-pulmonic consonants (i.e. those not made with lung air), and these are shown in Figure 2.2. These consonants are of three main types: clicks, implosives

Clicks		Voiced implosives		Ejectives	
⊙	Bilabial	ɓ	Bilabial	'	Examples:
ǀ	Dental	ɗ	Dental/alveolar	p'	Bilabial
ǃ	(Post)alveolar	ʄ	Palatal	t'	Dental/alveolar
ǂ	Palatoalveolar	ɠ	Velar	k'	Velar
ǁ	Alveolar lateral	ʛ	Uvular	s'	Alveolar fricative

Figure 2.2. Non-pulmonic consonant section of the IPA chart.

---

[8] [w] is placed among the 'other symbols' because its articulation involves simultaneous approximations of the articulators at two different places: bilabial and velar. Symbols for all such double articulations are placed in this part of the chart.

[9] [j] was chosen for this sound as the letter 'j' is used in such a way in many languages other than English, and ultimately derives from a version of Latin 'i' which stood for the approximant sound in that language. [j] is usually given the name 'yod' so we can distinguish the IPA symbol [j] from the letter 'y'.

and ejectives. None of these occurs linguistically in English (though all three types have been reported clinically as occurring in atypical speech, albeit rarely). Clicks can be found non-linguistically from English speakers as sounds of disapproval or encouragement (e.g. 'tut-tut' standing for the click [|], and the encouragement sound being the click [‖]).

To the right of this section we have the symbols for various suprasegmental features as seen in Figure 2.3. These include stress and length marks, both of which we may need to transcribe English; and tones and word accents. English is not a language that distinguishes words by the tones employed on them (unlike Chinese, for example), but we may need to mark intonation over longer stretches of speech (such as phrases), and symbols such as the ones shown in this section are often adapted for that purpose as well.

SUPRASEGMENTALS

ˈ	Primary stress	
ˌ	Secondary stress	
		ˌfoʊnəˈtɪʃən
ː	Long	eː
ˑ	Half-long	eˑ
̆	Extra-short	ĕ
|	Minor (foot) group	
‖	Major (intonation) group	
.	Syllable break	ɹi.ækt
‿	Linking (absence of a break)	

Figure 2.3. Suprasegmental section of the IPA chart.

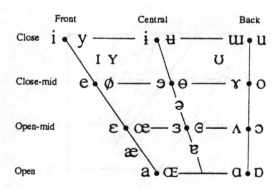

Figure 2.4. Vowel section of the IPA chart. Where symbols appear in pairs, the one to the right represents a rounded vowel.

Below this part of the chart we have the vowel diagram, reproduced in Figure 2.4. This is a conventional representation of the vowel area in the mouth (i.e. that part of the oral cavity where vowel sounds can be produced), with a series of vowel symbols provided which we can use to represent vowels in particular areas. Phoneticians have not always been happy that we can, impressionistically, make accurate estimates of the position of the articulators when we hear vowel sounds. Many, therefore, employ the Cardinal Vowel System (see Ball 1993 for more detail on this system). This is an auditory recognition system, where a series of cardinal vowels are learnt to be produced and recognized, and the vowels of natural language are classified in terms of how close they are to a particular cardinal value.

The vowel diagram on the IPA chart contains the symbols for the 18 cardinal vowels. These are the primary cardinal vowels [i, e, ε, a, ɑ, ɔ o, u], and the secondary cardinal vowels [y, ø, œ, Œ, ɒ, ʌ, ɤ, ɯ, ɨ, ʉ]. They are laid out in their traditional manner with their cardinal vowel numbers in Figures 2.5 and 2.6 below.

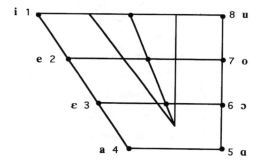

Figure 2.5. Primary cardinal vowels.

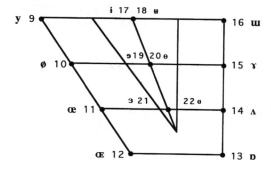

Figure 2.6. Secondary cardinal vowels.

Further central vowels have recently been added to the IPA version of the chart (cardinal vowels 19–22), and this also contains a series of symbols for what have been called 'lax' vowels, that is to say vowels that are pronounced without the articulators being at the boundaries of the vowel area, but relaxed more towards the centre. These vowels are common in many languages (including English), so it has proved useful to have special symbols for them ([ɪ, ʏ, ʊ, æ, ə, ɐ]).

We transcribe English vowels by adopting the symbol from the chart that is nearest in value to the particular English vowel in question. Only in a very detailed transcription (e.g. when transcribing a specific accent, or in clinical terms a disordered vowel system) do phoneticians add diacritics to vowel symbols in an attempt to show their precise quality. English accents may differ quite considerably in their vowel systems, and so we shall not list all the vowels needed to transcribe English vowels here. In a later section of this chapter we do give a few brief examples of English transcription, where the vowels of one accent are illustrated.

Diphthongs (that is to say vowel segments where the tongue glides from one position to another within the same syllable) are common in English, as in many languages. We transcribe them by using a symbol for the first part of the diphthong, and another for the last part. We can show they are diphthongs (rather than two vowels in different syllables next to each other) by using the linking diacritic: [aɪ] (as in English 'I'), but this linking mark is often omitted.

We have already mentioned the other symbols box briefly (see Figure 2.7). It contains the symbols for rare combinations of place and manner, or double articulations (such as [w]), and affricates such as [tʃ] and [dʒ], which we need to transcribe English 'ch'/'tch' and 'j'/'dge' respectively (as in 'church' and 'judge'). We normally omit the 'tie-bar' beneath the two symbols when transcribing English.

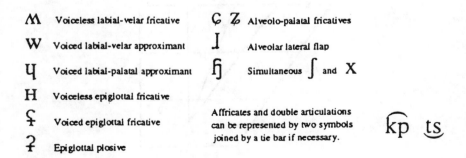

Figure 2.7. 'Other symbols' section of the IPA chart.

Finally, the chart contains a large box of diacritics, shown in Figure 2.8. These are marks that are added to consonant or vowel symbols to change the meaning of the symbol. Sometimes they represent slight differences in sound quality (such as a secondary articulation, as can be found in some English accents with [l] after a vowel where it becomes velarized: [ɫ]); in other instances the diacritic is used to avoid inventing a series of new

̥	Voiceless	n̥ d̥	̈	Breathy voiced	b̤ a̤	̪	Dental	t̪ d̪
̌	Voiced	s̬ t̬	̰	Creaky voiced	b̰ a̰	̺	Apical	t̺ d̺
ʰ	Aspirated	tʰ dʰ	̼	Linguolabial	t̼ d̼	̻	Laminal	t̻ d̻
̹	More rounded	ɔ̹	ʷ	Labialized	tʷ dʷ	̃	Nasalized	ẽ
̜	Less rounded	ɔ̜	ʲ	Palatalized	tʲ dʲ	ⁿ	Nasal release	dⁿ
̟	Advanced	u̟	ˠ	Velarized	tˠ dˠ	ˡ	Lateral release	dˡ
̠	Retracted	e̠	ˤ	Pharyngealized	tˤ dˤ	̚	No audible release	d̚
̈	Centralized	ë	˜	Velarized or pharyngealized	ɫ			
̽	Mid-centralized	e̽	̝	Raised	e̝	(ɹ̝ = voiced alveolar fricative)		
̩	Syllabic	n̩	̞	Lowered	e̞	(β̞ = voiced bilabial approximant)		
̯	Non-syllabic	e̯	̘	Advanced Tongue Root	e̘			
˞	Rhoticity	ɚ a˞	̙	Retracted Tongue Root	e̙			

Figure 2.8. Diacritics section of the IPA chart. Diacritics may be placed above a symbol with a descender, e.g. [ŋ̊]]

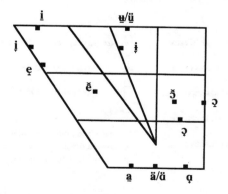

Figure 2.9. Use of diacritics with cardinal vowels.

symbols (such as the voiceless diacritic as used with the approximants: [l, l̥, ɹ, ɹ̥], etc. Diacritics need to be used with the cardinal vowel system so that the phonetician can illustrate how close to a particular cardinal vowel the vowel being described is. Figure 2.9 shows how specific vowel diacritics can be attached to cardinal vowel symbols, and in which part of the vowel diagram these combined symbols are to be plotted.

Many of these diacritics are important in transcribing disordered speech, so clinical phoneticians should ensure they learn how to use them from competent teachers and audio aids. We illustrate in the next chapter how to use some of them, along with extra diacritics and symbols especially for atypical sound types encountered in clinical situations.

How do we transcribe?

We have looked at what to transcribe, and the symbol system we need to do the transcribing. We also need to talk a little about how to undertake the actual transcription. It is possible to transcribe live: that is to say, to write down the transcription as the speaker is actually speaking. However, this becomes increasingly difficult the more detailed you want the transcription to be (see below), and for clinical phoneticians detailed transcriptions are normally required. If you want to transcribe suprasegmental features, and conversational aspects as well as segmental features, then a live transcription is probably impossible.

Nowadays, most phoneticians do their transcriptions from recorded data. Audiotape recordings can give excellent reproduction, as long as a good machine with an external microphone is used (see Tatham and Morton 1997 for fuller details about recording speech data). Many transcribers find, however, that much useful evidence to help in a transcription is lost if visual information is missing. Therefore, it is becoming more common to use videotaped material as well as audio. Visual information can help us in the transcription of lip-rounded vowels, or disambiguating unclear material (as is often found in clinical transcriptions). Videotape rarely gives a very good audio signal, however, so if you need clear audio (particularly if you intend to analyse the audio signal instrumentally) you should record via both video and audio recorders.

Once a suitable recording has been made, you need to ensure you have suitable playback facilities. This does not just mean good quality sound reproduction, but a machine that is capable of rewinding and replaying without having to depress the stop and play buttons. This is because you are bound to have to replay sections, one at a time, numerous times while you decide on the most appropriate consonant and vowel symbols and diacritics, and the relevant suprasegmental symbols. For particularly difficult or unclear passages, you may wish to have a tape loop constructed that will play the passage over and over again without having to use the rewind facility.[10]

Once you have finished transcribing, it is a good idea to make a clean copy of the entire transcription, and if you wish to keep a database of your material, to enter it into your computer. Nowadays, phonetic fonts are readily available for both IBM PC and Apple Macintosh formats, so there should be no trouble in computerizing your phonetic transcriptions.

If you are transcribing data for any kind of research project, you should ideally check your inter- and intra-scorer reliability. Inter-scorer reliability is checked by asking at least one other phonetically trained transcriber to undertake a transcription. This is then checked with your version, and percentage agreement of symbols is worked out (this can be done separately for consonants, vowels, diacritics, and suprasegmentals). If disagreements are found (as is almost always the case), the two scorers can listen together to the relevant sections, and see if they can reach agreement, though such changes should be noted in the research write-up. Remaining disagreements should also be noted.

Intra-scorer reliability assesses how consistent one particular transcriber is. To examine this, the transcriber repeats the transcription some days or weeks after it is first attempted. After this, a similar process of percentage agreement is undertaken as with the inter-scorer assessment. Again, any changes and remaining disagreements should be noted.

To conclude our discussion on phonetic transcription, we need to look in more depth at the difference between degrees of detail in transcription, and we address this in the next section.

Broad and narrow transcriptions

The terms 'broad' and 'narrow' are often applied to transcriptions to denote different amounts of detail that have been included. Although these terms are not strictly speaking the same as 'phonemic' and 'allophonic' transcriptions, the two sets of terms are often used interchangeably. A broad transcription is one that uses the simplest set of symbols and the smallest number of diacritics to transcribe a particular speech sample. This is often because the intended audience knows the precise value of the symbol owing to their phonetic knowledge of the language concerned. For example, a transcription of English aspirated [tʰ] as [t] in a broad transcription will not cause any ambiguity for a reader as

---

[10] If you have access to many of the computer-based acoustic analysis systems for speech (see Chapter 6) they can be set up to act as tape-loops for passages of your recording.

long as he or she knows that English [t] in certain word contexts is always aspirated. If a transcriber wishes to denote only the phonemes of a language, then the broad transcription can be termed a phonemic one, and symbols placed in slanted, rather than square, brackets. In this case our transcriber can use /t/ as a cover transcription for all the allophones of the /t/ phoneme. Broad transcriptions can also be used even if the intended readers are unlikely to know the precise phonetic values used if the aim of the transcription is to display only the broad characteristics of a language, or if it is being used to illustrate phonological rules operating at the phoneme level.

On the other hand, a narrow transcription is essential if the variety being described is not well known to the intended audience (such that they cannot disambiguate cover symbols such as /t/) or, indeed, is a novel variety not previously described. Disordered speech is, of course, always a novel variety, as it is unlikely that any two disordered speakers will have identical usage patterns. We return in Chapter 3 to the importance of narrow transcription of disordered data, but we can consider an example from natural language here. If the symbol /t/ is used in a phonemic transcription of English, then readers used only to British English varieties will be unaware that in word medial position in many American English varieties this symbol actually represents [ɾ] (an alveolar tap); whereas readers used only to American English varieties will be unaware that in word medial position in many British English accents this symbol actually represents [ʔ] (a glottal stop). Finally, both sets of readers will probably be unaware that in Hiberno-English varieties in word final position /t/ can actually stand for [θ̠] (a voiceless alveolar slit fricative).

Examples of transcriptions

In this section we present three transcriptions of the same passage: two phonemic transcriptions of Southern British Standard accent and a General American accent. The third transcription is a narrow transcription of the British accent. It should be noted that this narrow transcription does not display cardinal values for vowels, but does mark vowel nasalization and length where appropriate. The passage chosen is revisited in Chapter 7, where a transcription of a disfluent speaker is examined.

The passage is shown first in ordinary orthography:

The World Cup Finals of 1982 are held in Spain this year. They will involve the top nations of the world in a tournament lasting over four weeks held at fourteen different centres in Spain. All of the first round games will be in the provincial towns, with the semi-finals and final held in Barcelona and Madrid.

SBS phonemic transcription

/ðə ˈwɜːld ˈkʌp ˈfaɪnl̩z əv ˈnaɪntin eɪti ˈtu ə ˈheld ɪn ˈspeɪn ðɪʃ ˈjɜ. ðeɪ wɪl ɪnˈvɒlv ðə ˈtɒp ˈneɪʃn̩z əv ðə ˈwɜːld ɪn ə ˈtʊənəmənt ˈlɑstɪŋ əʊvə ˈfɔ ˈwiks ˈheld ət ˈfɔtin ˈdɪfrənt ˈsentəz ɪn ˈspeɪn. ɔl əv ðə ˈfɜst ˈraʊnd ˈgeɪmz wɪl bi ɪn ðə prəˈvɪnʃl̩ ˈtaʊnz wɪð ðə ˈsemifaɪnl̩z əŋ ˈfaɪnl̩ ˈheld ɪm bɑsɪˈləʊnə əm ˈmədrɪd/

General American transcription

/ðə ˈwɚld ˈkʌp ˈfaɪnl̩z əv ˈnaɪntin eɪɾi ˈtu ɚ ˈheld ɪn ˈspeɪn ðɪʃ ˈjɚ. ðeɪ wɪl ɪnˈvɑlv ðə ˈtɑp ˈneɪʃn̩z əv ðə ˈwɚld ɪn ə ˈtɚrnəmənt ˈlæstɪŋ oʊvɚ ˈfor ˈwiks ˈheld ət ˈfortin ˈdɪfərənt ˈsentɚz ɪn ˈspeɪn. ɔl əv ðə ˈfɚst ˈraʊnd ˈgeɪmz wɪl bi ɪn ðə prəˈvɪnʃl̩ ˈtaʊnz wɪð ðə ˈsemaɪfaɪnl̩z əŋ ˈfaɪnl̩ ˈheld ɪm bɑrsəˈloʊnə əm ˈmədrɪd/

SBS narrow transcription

[ð̥ə ˈwɜːtd̥ ˈkʰʌpˈ ˈfaɪ̃n̩t̮z̥ əɣ ˈnãɪ̃nt̪ʰin eɪt̪ʰi ˈt̪ʰuː ə ˈhetd̥ ˈɪn ˈsp̈eɪ̃n ð̥ɪʃ ˈjɜː. ð̥eɪ wɪt ɪnˈɣɒtɣ ð̥ə ˈt̪ʰɒpˈ ˈneɪʃn̩z̥ əɣ ð̥ə ˈwɜːtd̥ ˈɪn ə ˈt̪ʰʊ̃ə̃n̪ə̃mə̃ntˈ ˈlɑːst̪ʊ̃ŋ əʊvə ˈfɔː ˈwiːks ˈhetd̥ ət ˈfɔːt̪ʰin ˈd̥ɪfɹ̩ə̃ntˈ ˈsẽnt̪ʰəz̥ ˈɪn ˈsp̈eɪ̃n. ɔːt əɣ ð̥ə ˈfɜːstˈ ˈɹ̩aʊ̃d̥ ˈg̊eɪ̃mz wɪt b̥i ˈɪn ð̥ə pɹ̩əˈɣɪ̃nʃt ˈt̪ʰaʊ̃z wɪð̥ ð̥ə ˈsẽmifaɪ̃n̩t̮z̥ ə̃ŋ ˈfaɪ̃n̩t ˈhetd̥ ˈɪm b̥ɑːsɪˈləʊ̃nə ə̃m ˈməd̥ɹ̩ɪd̥]

Further reading

To understand phonetic symbols you will need to know about articulatory phonetics, as the labels used on the IPA chart mostly derive from traditional terms in that branch of the science. Any good introduction to phonetics will give this, for example Laver (1994), Clark and Yallop (1995), Ladefoged (1993), Ball and Rahilly (1999), and especially designed for speech-language pathologists, Ball (1993). The history of transcription can be found in Abercrombie (1967) and in Ball, Rahilly and Tench (1996).

Information about recording and displaying speech is given in Tatham and Morton (1997), while the problems of scorer reliability is discussed in some depth in Shriberg and Lof (1991). Finally, more discussion of the difference between broad and narrow transcriptions is given in Ball, Rahilly and Tench (1996).

CHAPTER 3

Transcribing Disordered Speech

In the previous chapter we examined phonetic transcription, and how best to go about making a transcription of speech data. We return here to disordered speech, and look at the specific problems raised by the need to transcribe data of this sort. This does not affect transcribing technique as much as the transcription tools at our disposal. As we have seen, the International Phonetic Alphabet (IPA) is the best available tool for phonetic transcription, whether we are interested in broad phonemic aspects of speech, or narrower phonetic aspects. Of course, in looking at disordered speech, we are not justified in adopting a broad or phonemic type of description. This is because the fact that the speaker is disordered phonologically means that they are not using an accepted phonological (or phonemic) system. We need, therefore, to adopt an approach that aims to include in our transcription as much phonetic detail as we are able to distinguish, as we do not know at an early stage of analysis what aspects of the client's speech will prove to be important in phonological assessment and remediation.

In this chapter, therefore, we shall be looking at what extra symbolization we need to cope with transcribing atypical speech, and the dangers of inadequate transcription, and we shall provide illustrations of transcriptions of different types of speech disorder.

Symbolizing atypical speech

As we saw in the last chapter, the IPA provides a wide range of symbols to help in the transcribing of natural language. Unfortunately, however, the clinical phonetician may well be faced with the task of transcribing some sounds that do not occur in natural language, or are so rare that no IPA symbol or diacritic is available. Until recently, clinical phoneticians had to rely on *ad hoc* additions to the symbol set to deal with such sounds, or to adopt localized traditions with no international currency (see, for example, discussion in Ball 1993, Ball, Rahilly and Tench 1996, Duckworth *et al* 1990). In the 1980s there developed a move to provide an internationally recognized set of symbols as an extension to the IPA to enable clinical phoneticians to transcribe disordered and atypical speech in detail. The first of these developments (the PRDS symbols) was superseded and expanded by the extIPA symbols drawn up in 1989, and most recently modified in 1994 (see the previous references for further details of these developments). The abbreviation 'extIPA' stands for the 'Extensions to the IPA for the transcription of disordered speech', and the extIPA symbols are set out on a chart in a similar fashion to the IPA symbols. Just as we did in the last chapter, we shall look at the extIPA chart in its several sections.

The main part of the extIPA chart is the consonants chart at the top, and this is reproduced in Figure 3.1. This contains symbols for consonants not on the normal IPA chart, but apart from that is laid out in a similar fashion. The columns across the top are labelled in terms of place of articulation (and as in the IPA chart these follow the tradition of the leftmost rows relating to places of articulation furthest forward in the mouth, getting progressively further back the further right you move). The rows down the side are manners of articulation (again generally following the tradition of moving from consonants involving oral closure at the top of the chart, to more open manners at the bottom). Further, where appropriate, symbols at the left in a box are voiceless, while those on the right are voiced. This chart also has shaded boxes to show impossible articulations, and boxes that are left empty either because a normal IPA symbol is used for those

	bilabial	labiodental	dentolabial	labioalv.	linguolabial	interdental	bidental	alveolar	velar	velophar.
Plosive		p̪ b̪	p̄ b̄	p̞ b̞	t̼ d̼	t̪ d̪				
Nasal			m̄	m̞	n̼	n̪				
Trill					r̼	r̪				
Fricative median			f̄ v̄	f̠ v̠	θ̼ ð̼	θ̪ ð̪	ɦ̪ ɦ̪			fŋ
Fricative lateral+median								ʪ ʫ		
Fricative nareal	m̃							ñ̰	ŋ̃	
Percussive	w̥ w						ʬ			
Approximant lateral					l̼	l̪				

Figure 3.1. Consonant section of the extIPA chart (revised to 1997).

sounds, or when no symbol is needed because the sound is so rare in both natural language and atypical speech.

The consonant symbols provided on this chart are for sounds that are reported sufficiently often to the various panels responsible for drawing up sets of symbols for atypical speech that it was felt worthwhile to provide a symbol for them. It should be noted that clinical phoneticians may often come across occasional usage of sounds that are not dealt with by the extIPA system. After a time, however, it becomes impractical to provide a symbol for every rare sound encountered. The extIPA set is an attempt to find a compromise between the demands for symbols for every possible sound, and the desire to keep the number of new symbols to be learnt to an absolute minimum. As we shall demonstrate later in this chapter, imprecise phonetic transcriptions can sometimes be worse than none at all, but there is a price to pay in reliability the more symbols that are available.

The places of articulation on this consonant chart are a mixture of ones that are familiar from the ordinary IPA chart, and novel ones. These latter include dentolabial (sometimes referred to as reverse labio-dental), where the articulation is between the upper lip and the lower front teeth, labioalveolar where the articulation is between the lower lip and the alveolar ridge (found with speakers with excessive overbite for target bilabial and labiodental sounds), and bidental where the articulation is between the upper and lower teeth. Linguolabial is also on the chart despite the relevant diacritic being included on the main IPA chart. The reason for this is that this articulation is very rare in natural language, but relatively frequent in clinical data perhaps as a realization of target alveolars; the chart therefore illustrates the diacritic on a range of consonant types. Interdental articulation is not separately recognized from dental on the IPA chart: dental and interdental fricatives are assumed to be slight variations that may occur from speaker to speaker in languages that have these sounds. However, in clinical phonetics we may well need to note a consistent use of interdental articulations (i.e. with tongue tip protrusion) for target apical sounds, and the extIPA extension of the IPA dental diacritic to show this is very useful. Finally, we can note the inclusion of the velopharyngeal place of articulation: that is to say articulation at the velopharyngeal port. We shall return to this sound type below.

The manners of articulation rows are generally those of the IPA chart; however, three new types are included. Fricatives are generally thought of as being either median with airflow over the centre of the tongue (such as [s], [θ], [ʃ]) or lateral with airflow down one or both sides of the tongue (as in [ɬ], [ɮ]). However, it is possible to produce fricatives with airflow both centrally through a small groove down the middle of the tongue, and laterally through a small gap at the side of the tongue, and such sounds have been reported clinically. Therefore, the extIPA chart provides symbols to transcribe such lateral and median fricatives: the symbols are designed to remind the user of the central and lateral aspects of the sounds.

A second new type of fricative is where the friction is located within the nasal cavity at the nares (nostrils), and can be thought of as nasals with audible turbulent airflow through the nose. A diacritic is provided to denote these sounds adapted from the normal nasal tilde mark with the addition of two dots to represent the nares, and as we shall see can also be added to any other sounds that have this added nareal friction. Finally, we have the percussive manner type. Like the last two types, this is not reported for natural language, but is made by bringing together sharply and briefly two moveable articulators (or possible one moveable and one static articulator). Both bidental percussives (banging together of the upper and lower teeth) and bilabial percussives have been reported, and the symbols adopted attempt to show the binary nature of these sounds.

The other symbols in this part of the chart are mostly based on IPA consonants with added diacritics. So labiodental plosives have the dental diacritic added to labial symbols; the dentolabials have the dental diacritic added above the symbol instead of below, and the interdentals have the diacritic both above and below the symbol. The bidental fricative uses the same diacritic placement as the interdentals, but as they are placed on the symbols for the glottal fricatives ([h], [ɦ]) it is understood these sounds have no tongue tip involvement, and are in fact fricatives made through clenched teeth.

As noted above, the linguolabials make use of an IPA diacritic (supposed to remind us of a lip shape), but the labioalveolar uses a new diacritic. The IPA has no diacritic for alveolar place of articulation, which can be thought of as a problem. We may often wish to note for natural language that a particular articulation is alveolar as opposed to dental (e.g. for the slit-t of Irish English which is an alveolar non-grooved fricative). For disordered speech this may be more important, and for this combined labioalveolar articulation is clearly a necessity. The extIPA symbols therefore include a subscript equals sign for alveolar, and to denote labioalveolars this is added to the labial symbols.

Finally, we have one other new symbol: the velopharyngeal fricative (sometimes called the velopharyngeal snort). This is shown by a symbol derived from a combination of a fricative ([f]) and a velar nasal ([ŋ]), but is intended to be a single symbol, and not a sequence.

↔ labial spreading	s̳	ǁ strong articulation	f̬	∼ denasal	m̃
ˮ dentolabial	v̂	˧ weak articulation	v̰	˜ nasal escape	ṽ
ˮ interdental/bidental	n̟	\ reiterated articulation	p\p\p	≁ velopharyngeal friction	s̃
= alveolar	l̳	⁺ whistled articulation	s̟	↓ ingressive airflow	p↓
˗ linguolabial	d̳	→ sliding articulation	θs̪	↑ egressive airflow	!↑

Figure 3.2. Diacritic section of the extIPA chart.

Beneath the main consonant chart is the box for diacritics, and this is shown in Figure 3.2. Some of these we have already encountered on the main chart (dentolabial, interdental/bidental, labiolingual, nasal escape/nareal friction), while others are new. Some of these fill in gaps on the IPA (e.g. a lip-spreading diacritic to complement the lip rounding diacritic; alveolar to complement the dental and post-dental positions; denasal to complement the nasal diacritic), but others are specifically for atypical speech: strong and weak articulations, reiterated articulation (as in stuttering), whistled fricatives, and sliding articulation (i.e. rapid movement of the articulators from one position to another within the time frame of a single segment). The double tilde mark is the diacritic to show simultaneous velopharyngeal friction with any sound (see above for the velopharyngeal fricative by itself), and the upward and downward arrows can be used to illustrate direction of airflow. This last will be most useful when transcribing pulmonic ingressive speech, for which the IPA has had no symbol, but which is comparatively commonly reported in clinical data.

Beneath the diacritics box there are two further boxes of symbols, dealing with connected speech and with voicing. The IPA has generally avoided recommending symbols for transcribing aspects of connected speech such as pauses, tempo and loudness. However, as these aspects are often important in disordered speech, the extIPA system includes them (see Figure 3.3) in an attempt to bring some consistency to their symbolization, as a plethora of competing systems have been used in the past (see Ball, Rahilly and Tench 1996). The symbols proposed for pauses are periods (full stops) within parentheses. The parentheses mark the periods as being connected speech phenomena, rather than the IPA diacritic that marks hiatus between vowels. For pauses longer than a second or so (such as may be encountered in dysfluent or aphasic speech), the length of time in seconds is entered within the parentheses (e.g. (6 seconds)).

(.)	short pause
(..)	medium pause
(...)	long pause
f	loud speech [{*f* lɑʊd *f*}]
ff	louder speech [{*ff* lɑʊdə· *ff*}]
p	quiet speech [{*p* kwaɪət *p*}]
pp	quieter speech [{*pp* kwaɪətə *pp*}]
allegro	fast speech [{*allegro* fɑːst *allegro*}]
lento	slow speech [{ *lento* slou *lento*}]
crescendo, ralentando, etc may also be used	

Figure 3.3. Connected speech section of the extIPA chart.

The musical notation adopted for tempo and loudness is mostly self-evident and widely encountered in studies of conversation. The novel aspect is the use of the curly braces to show over which stretch of speech the particular tempo or loudness is operating. This allows us to integrate segmental symbols (i.e. the vowels and consonants) with suprasegmental symbols (i.e. those operating over a stretch of vowels and consonants) within the same transcription. As we shall see below, we can use this approach for transcribing voice quality as well.

In Figure 3.4 we show the diacritics that can be used for very detailed transcription of phonatory activity. With these extra diacritics we can show

- whether a sound is completely or only partially voiced or voiceless
- if partially, whether voicing or devoicing is present at the initial or final part of the segment
- whether pre- or post-voicing occurs
- whether a sound is aspirated or unaspirated or pre-aspirated.

Although such detail may be difficult to detect without instrumental analysis (see Chapter 6), it acts as a useful means of recording the findings of such an analysis and incorporating them into your transcription. Voicing difficulties are reported in a wide range of speech disorders, so clinical phoneticians may well need to make use of this system.

The final part of the extIPA chart consists of a series of 'other' symbols, mostly to help in the transcription of indeterminate sounds. Transcribers may find sounds indeterminate because of the quality of the tape, background noise, or simply because the sound is so unusual they are unable to find a description for it.

However, in such cases, we may well have some idea as to the kind of sound(s) that are causing problems: we may feel certain a sound is a

ˬ	pre-voicing	ˬz
ˬ	post-voicing	zˬ
₍̥₎	partial devoicing	₍z̥₎
₍̥	initial partial devoicing	₍z̥
̥₎	final partial devoicing	z̥₎
₍ˬ₎	partial voicing	₍s̬₎
₍ˬ	initial partial voicing	₍s̬
ˬ₎	final partial voicing	s̬₎
=	unaspirated	p=
ʰ	pre-aspiration	ʰp

Figure 3.4. Phonatory activity diacritic section of the extIPA chart.

(̄) indeterminate sound	(()) extraneous noise ((2 sylls))
(V̄), (P̄l) indeterminate vowel, plosive, etc	¡ sublaminal lower alveolar percussive click
(P̄l,vls) indeterminate voiceless plosive, etc	!¡ alveolar & sublaminal click ('cluck-click')
() silent articulation (ʃ), (m)	* sound with no available symbol

Figure 3.5. 'Other symbols' section of the extIPA chart.

consonant rather than a vowel, or a fricative rather than a plosive, or that it is voiced rather than voiceless, or bilabial rather than at any other place of articulation. The system of indeterminacy included on the extIPA chart allows the clinical phonetician to record as much (or as little) as they are sure about with a balloon or circle (printed as two parentheses joined at the top and bottom by straight lines). The examples on the chart show, therefore, how different degrees of indeterminacy are recorded within these balloons.

Among the remaining symbols is one to allow us to transcribe silent articulations or 'zero-airstream' (i.e. 'mouthing', when a speaker moves the articulators into position to make a sound but no airstream is activated, resulting in silence). Clearly this is different from the deletion of the sound altogether, and deserves to be recorded separately, though it has to be recognized that it is easy to do this only with target bilabials, and even then we are guessing which particular segment the speaker may have been attempting. The last few symbols cover a means of noting extraneous noise within a transcription (e.g. a dog barking, or door slamming), and sounds that are recognized, but for which no symbol is currently available (which can be described in a footnote after the transcription). Two types of unusual click are also symbolized.

The extIPA system, therefore, gives a range of extra symbols thus allowing the clinical transcriber to deal with a wide range of atypical speech at both the segmental and suprasegmental levels. It does not, however, deal with the complex area of voice quality and voice disorders, for which we need to investigate the VoQS system.

Symbolizing voice quality

To transcribe voice quality, both normal and disordered, we recommend the VoQS system as described in Ball, Esling and Dickson (1999). This system too uses curly braces to enclose the stretch of speech over which a particular voice quality operates, with various voice quality symbols attached to the braces.

The voice quality symbols are divided into those connected with the airstream, those dependent on phonation type, and those derived from particular supralaryngeal (or articulatory) settings. Some of these may occur together, of course, as (for example) a velarized supralaryngeal setting could be used at the same time as whisper phonation. Most of the symbols used for the various voice types are derived from IPA and extIPA diacritics, or the symbols suggested in Laver (1980), and an example of how they are used is given at the foot of the chart. The VoQS chart is given in Figure 3.6, and also in the charts appendix at the end of the book.

This example also shows that different degrees of a voice quality can be noted through the use of numerals (1–3 being the recommended range). However, we must be careful as to what is implied by the use of a voice quality symbol. For example, if whisper or creak is noted for a stretch of speech, it does not mean that every sound is uttered on that phonation type; rather, that normally voiced sounds are pronounced with this phonation type, while normally voiceless ones remain voiceless. Otherwise, speakers would not be able to maintain the contrast between target voiced and voiceless sounds. Likewise, if we use the velarized voice symbol, it implies that there is a tendency (the use of numerals can note how strong that tendency is) to raise the back of the tongue towards the velum during speech (except with velar sounds of course). Finally, we can consider the nasal voice quality symbol. If we attach this to a stretch of speech we are signalling that there is a tendency to keep the velum from being fully raised during target non-nasals; again, the numerals can mark how strong the resultant nasality is.

Airstream types

Œ	oesophageal speech	И	electrolarynx speech
Ю	tracheo-oesophageal speech	↓	pulmonic ingressive speech

Phonation types

V	modal voice	F	falsetto
W	whisper	C	creak
V̤	whispery voice (murmur)	V̰	creaky voice
Ç	whispery creak	V!	harsh voice
V!!	ventricular phonation	V̰!!	diplophonia
V̬	anterior or pressed phonation	W̲	posterior whisper

Supralaryngeal settings

L̝	raised larynx	L̞	lowered larynx
Vᵒᵉ	labialized voice (open round)	Vʷ	labialized voice (close round)
V̚	spread-lip voice	Vᵛ	labio-dentalized voice
V̺	linguo-apicalized voice	V̻	linguo-laminalized voice
V˞	retroflex voice	V̪	dentalized voice
V̲	alveolarized voice	V̲ʲ	palatoalveolarized voice
Vʲ	palatalized voice	Vˠ	velarized voice
Vʁ	uvularized voice	Vˁ	pharyngealized voice
V̰ˁ	laryngo-pharyngealized voice	Vᴴ	faucalized voice
Ṽ	nasalized voice	V̓	denasalized voice
J̞	open jaw voice	J̝	close jaw voice
J̬	right offset jaw voice	J̭	left offset jaw voice
J̟	protruded jaw voice	Θ	protruded tongue voice

Use of labelled braces and numerals to mark stretches of speech and
degrees and combinations of voice quality

['ðɪs ɪz 'nɔˑməl 'vɔɪs {3V! 'ðɪs ɪz 'veɹɪ 'hɑˑʃ 'vɔɪs 3V!} 'ðɪs ɪz 'nɔˑməl 'vɔɪs
wʌns 'mɔˑ {L̝1V! 'ðɪs ɪz 'les 'hɑˑʃ 'vɔɪs wɪð 'louəd 'læɹɪŋks 1V!L̝}]

Figure 3.6. Voice quality symbols: VoQS chart.

Broad and narrow transcription (revisited)

In Chapter 2 we discussed the difference between a broad and a narrow transcription, and the importance of giving as much detail as possible within a clinical transcription. We have just reviewed the additional symbol systems for disordered segmental and suprasegmental aspects of speech. However, if we decide not to use these, and to use only very broad transcriptions of data, what sort of problems arise? In this section, we shall take a brief look at how we can both underestimate and overestimate the phonological and phonetic abilities of client's speech if we do not record sufficient detail. To illustrate this we shall use examples first recorded in Ball, Rahilly and Tench (1996).

The first of these examples compares a broad and narrow transcription of the same set of data from a speech disordered subject. Both transcriptions are set in square brackets, for although one of them is more detailed than the other, neither is a phonemic transcription, if only because disordered phonology of itself cannot be representative of the target phonological system.

Speaker B. Age 6;9. Broad transcription

pin	[pɪn]	ten	[ten]
bin	[pɪn]	den	[ten]
cot	[kɑːt]	pea	[piː]
got	[kɑːt]	bee	[piː]

This data set suggests that there is a collapse of phonological contrast: specifically, the contrast between voiced and voiceless plosives in word-initial position. This clearly leads to homonymic clashes between, for example, 'pin' and 'bin' and 'cot' and 'got' respectively. As word-initial plosives have a high functional load in English, such a loss of voicing contrast in this context clearly requires treatment.

However, if a narrow transcription of the same data is examined, the picture alters.

Speaker B. Age 6;9. Narrow transcription

pin	[pʰɪn]	ten	[tʰen]
bin	[pɪn]	den	[ten]
cot	[kʰɑːt]	pea	[pʰiː]
got	[kɑːt]	bee	[piː]

It is clear from this transcription that there is not, in fact, a loss of contrast between initial voiced and voiceless plosives. Target voiceless plosives are realized without vocal fold vibration (voice), but with aspiration on release (as are the adult target forms). The target voiced plosives are realized without aspiration (as with the adult forms), but also without any vocal fold vibration. It is this last difference that distinguishes them from the target form. For, although adult English 'voiced' plosives are often devoiced for some of their duration in initial position, totally voiceless examples are rare.

Ball *et al* note that although insufficiently narrow phonetic description can often underestimate the disordered client's phonological ability, it can also sometimes overestimate it. This may occur when the transcriber is limited to the symbols used in a phonemic transcription of English, or where they are influenced by the expected sound (or both). We show below the sample from speaker D of Ball, Rahilly and Tench (1996).

Speaker D. Age 7;2. Broad transcription

mat	[mæt͡s]	pat	[pæt͡s]
top	[t͡sɑːp]	tin	[t͡sɪn]
match	[mæt͡ʃ]	patch	[pæt͡ʃ]
chop	[t͡ʃɑːp]	chin	[t͡ʃɪn]

This transcription suggests that the speaker maintains a contrast between target /t/ and /tʃ/. The affricate appears to be pronounced as the adult target, whereas the plosive is realized as an affricate at the alveolar place of articulation. However, if we examine the narrow transcription, we can see that in this instance, a restriction to the symbols used in transcribing adult English has led to an overestimation of this patient's abilities:

Speaker D. Age 7;2. Narrow transcription

mat	[mæt͡ʂ]	pat	[pæt͡ʂ]
top	[t͡ʂɑːp]	tin	[t͡ʂɪn]
match	[mæt͡ʂ]	patch	[pæt͡ʂ]
chop	[t͡ʂɑːp]	chin	[t͡ʂɪn]

This speaker in fact uses a retroflex affricate for both target /t/ and /tʃ/. The expected alveolar and post-alveolar positions appear to have influenced the choice of symbols in the first transcription. The more detailed second transcription does demonstrate that the contrast between these phonemes is lost, and will need to be re-established in therapy.

Transcription reliability

There are, however, problems with narrow transcriptions. Studies show that the more detailed a transcription is required to be, the less reliable it is likely to be. One of the most important studies in this area is that undertaken by Shriberg and Lof (1991), who looked at inter-scorer and intra-scorer reliability in narrow phonetic transcription of clinical speech data. They looked at a wide range of features that could affect reliability in transcription (such as severity of speech disorder, the position within the word of the segment, broad versus narrow transcription, etc.). Among their numerous conclusions was that narrow transcription was about 20% less reliable than broad (though reliability even here was around 75%). They recommended that with detailed descriptions of clinical data transcription should be aided by the use of instrumental analysis (such techniques as are described in Chapters 4–9 of this book).

Ball and Rahilly (1996) describe one such example in detail. The authors were attempting a detailed impressionistic transcription of a taped sample of stuttered speech. Not only was the stutter severe, with numerous repetitions, but there were also changes in voice quality (including both breathy and creaky voice), velopharyngeal fricatives, pulmonic ingressive speech, quiet speech and strong articulations. As well as the problem of transcribing these features, there was the added difficulty that the transcribers were working from an old tape that had a considerable amount of background noise.

Nevertheless, the authors demonstrated that acoustic analysis of the passage allowed the transcription of the whole piece with a fair degree of confidence. This kind of analysis was particularly useful during passages of very quiet repetition, where a spectrogram (see Chapter 6) allowed the transcribers to calculate the number of repetitions involved at specific points. The authors noted that their exercise in analysis had demonstrated how useful the acoustic record can be in resolving problematic aspects of phonetic transcription. We can also use articulatory instrumental analysis, of course, and we return to that area in Chapters 4 and 5.

Examples of transcriptions of clinical data

In this section we shall illustrate some of the speech disorders described in Chapter 1 by providing transcriptions of representative speech samples. These transcriptions are narrow, and make use of the symbols of the IPA, extIPA and VoQS where appropriate. Many of these examples are adapted from Ball, Rahilly and Tench (1996).

Example 1

The child in this example has a general fronting process which results in some phonemic substitution patterns, but others where atypical sounds are utilized.

thin	[θ̬ɪn̬]	so	[s̬oʊ]
cat	[tæt̬]	foot	[ɸʊt̬]
shop	[sɑːp]	dog	[d̬ɑːd]
both	[boʊθ̬]	tease	[ti̬ːz̬]
that	[ð̬æt]	goose	[duːs̬]

The fronting does not result, however, in the loss of phonemic contrastivity, although the speech sounds very disturbed.

Example 2

This child exhibits what is commonly termed a lisp. However, the detailed transcription shows that two distinct lisp types are exhibited, which again maintain phonological contrastivity.

sip	[ɬɪp]	zip	[ʒɪp]
hiss	[hɪɬ]	his	[hɪʒ]
racer	[ɹeɪɬɚ]	razor	[ɹeɪʒɚ]
stop	[ɬtɑːp]	lost	[lɑːɬt]
spy	[ɬpaɪ]	buzzed	[bʌʒd]
ship	[ʃɪp]	hush	[hʌʃ]
pressure	[pɹeʃɚ]	pleasure	[pleʒɚ]
wished	[wɪʃt]	garage	[ɡəɹɑːʒ]

Target alveolar fricatives are realized as alveolar lateral fricatives, but target palato-alveolars are realized as combined median and lateral fricatives. Auditorily, these may sound very similar, but it is clear the child does maintain a phonological contrast.

Example 3

This case concerns the overuse of a lip-shape harmonization process. Here, alveolar contexts produce a lip-spreading process, while labial, palato-alveolar and velar contexts produce a lip-rounding process. These processes affect both consonants and vowels.

ten	[ten]	two	[tɯː]
nod	[nɑːd]	loose	[lɯːs]

peep	[pyːp]	keep	[kʷyːp]
beam	[byːm]	gang	[gʷœŋʷ]
sheep	[ʃʷyːp]	rip	[ɹʷʏp]

When both alveolar and non-alveolar sounds are present in the word, progressive assimilation is seen:

tube	[tyːb]	dog	[dɑːg]
sheet	[ʃʷyːtʷ]	read	[ɹʷyːdʷ]
green	[gʷɹʷyːnʷ]	bead	[byːdʷ]

Clearly, this case is quite complex, and the child seems unable to divorce the lip-posture from the place of articulation.

Example 4

The data for this case are adapted from Howard (1993).

baby	[b̃eɪbɪ]	toy	[ʔɔɪ]
cat	[ʔæʔʰ]	tap	[ʔæʔʘ]
paper	[p̃eɪp̃ʔə]	kick	[ʔɪʔʰ]
bucket	[b̃ʊʔɪʔʰ]	Sue	[ç̃u]
Daddy	[ʔæʔɪ]	dog	[ʔɒʔʰ]
sugar	[ç̃ɬʊʔə]	shoe	[ç̃ʷu]

These data are taken from a child with cleft palate, and illustrate the child's realization of place contrasts. It is interesting that, although these pronunciations are often markedly deviant from the target, they manage in many cases to maintain contrastivity. So, although alveolars are most often realized by glottal stops for plosives, bilabials retain some kind of bilabial aspects. Velars, however, are not regularly distinguished from alveolars. The following data also show that alveolar and palato-alveolar targets are usually contrasted, as are plosives, fricatives and affricates, as well as approximants, at least in word-initial position.

tap	[ʔæʔʘ]	down	[ʔaʊɴ]
chair	[ʔjɛə]	jam	[ʔjæm]
sock	[ç̃ɒʔʰ]	shop	[ç̃ʷjɒp̃ʰ]
zip	[ç̃ɪʔʘ]	cup	[ʔʊʔʰ]
go	[ʔəʊ]	yes	[jɛʔ]
why	[waɪ]	letter	[ɰeʔə]
glasses	[ɴwæç̃ə̃ç̃]	ring	[ʊɪɴ]

The nasal–oral contrast was usually maintained, though again not often according to the target norms. In fact, the following data demonstrate that a uvular nasal is used for both alveolar and velar nasal targets (bilabial nasals having been satisfactorily established during therapy) in contrast to the glottal stop or bilabial plosives (again these latter having been worked on in therapy) used for the oral stops.

letter	[ɰeʔə]	nose	[nəʊɢ̃]
ladder	[ɰæʔə]	ring	[ʊɪɴ]
sugar	[ɕ̃ɭʊʔə]	fine	[f̃ːaɪɴ]
down	[ʔaʊɴ]	penny	[p̃ʔenɪ]
dog	[ʔɒʔʰ]	singing	[ɕ̃ɪnɪɴ]
cat	[ʔæʔʰ]	teaspoon	[ʔĩɕ̃ bʊɴ]
pig	[ɔɪʔʰ]	mud	[məʔʰ]
pen	[ʔeɴ]	mum	[məm]
tap	[ʔæʔɵ]	mouth	[maʊθ]
paper	[p̃ʔeɪpə]	thumb	[θəm]
big	[mɪʔʰ]	jam	[ʔjæm]
baby	[b̃eɪbɪ]	hammer	[h̃æmə]

These data also demonstrate the child's general success with the dental fricatives.

This case shows markedly deviant pronunciations, but also the importance of accurate and detailed transcriptions – not only to demonstrate the articulatory strategies adopted by this particular subject, but also to highlight those areas where contrastivity is maintained and those where it is lost.

Example 5

The data for this case are adapted from Ball *et al* (1994). In the transcript, 'T' stands for the therapist, and 'W' for the patient.

T: just ask you to say a few phrases . . . open the door
W: [{*lento* Ṽ !! oʊʔən ə d̪eː Ṽ !! *lento*}]
T: close the window
W: [{*lento* Ṽ !! hloʊh ə wɪnd̪oʊ Ṽ !! *lento*}]
T: wash the dishes
W: [{*lento* Ṽ !! wɒh ə ʔɪhɪhɪː Ṽ !! *lento*}]

Subject W is a dysarthric patient, and we can note from the transcription the use of weakly articulated segments, deletion of certain initial sounds, and a weakening of fricatives to [h]. As is often the case with dysarthria, there is what can be termed a pervasive lenition in operation which has been shown through the use of the weak articulation diacritic.

Finally, we can note that a transcription of a disfluent speaker is given and explained in Chapter 7.

Further reading

Further examples of how broad transcriptions can provide misleading data are given in Carney (1979). Ball, Rahilly and Tench (1996) provide a large sample of transcriptions of types of disordered speech, and also show how the extended IPA symbols for the transcription of atypical speech are used. The background to the development of the extIPA symbols is given in Duckworth *et al* (1990).

CHAPTER 4

Articulatory Instrumentation

The articulatory aspects of phonetics cover speech production from the initiation of an airstream through to the emitting of sound through the oral and/or nasal cavities. Most of the stages in the speech production process can be investigated through instrumental means, and in this chapter we shall look at the most common and most useful of these techniques. Some of the instrumentation we shall discuss is expensive and not accessible to all clinical phoneticians, but more and more experimental phonetic techniques are becoming user-friendly and available through personal computer packages. It is, therefore, valuable for clinical phoneticians and speech language pathologists to become aware of these approaches, and prepared to use them when they get that opportunity.

Muscle activity

If we now take the stages of speech production one by one, we can then note what sort of instrumentation is available for each of these stages. First, we can consider the neurophonetic stages that come into play after the linguistic aspects of an utterance have been planned. Various brain scanning techniques are available that can be used to examine neurological activity connected with speech (and we shall mention some of these briefly below); however, phoneticians have probably been more concerned with investigating the results of such planning: that is to say, muscle activity. Electrical activity in the muscles of speech has been examined by phoneticians through a technique called electromyography (EMG). This technique requires the placing of small electrodes in or over the muscles of interest, and the recording of the electrical activity going on there; this can then be synchronized with a recording of the speech involved, and so muscle contractions can be viewed in conjunction with the speech signal.

41

For some muscles that are near the surface of the skin, surface electrodes can be used that are simply attached by a special adhesive to the skin above the muscle. Investigations of the lip muscle (*orbicularis oris*) have been undertaken in this fashion. Other muscles need the use of needle electrodes or hooked wire electrodes that are placed directly into the muscle. Some laryngeal muscles have been investigated in this way.

EMG has proved a very useful tool in the investigation of muscle activity in both normal and disordered speech and, as with many of the techniques described in this chapter, has been used both as an analytic/diagnostic technique and as a form of feedback to patients to enable them to correct speech patterns.

Initiation

Muscle activity is of course required for all movements of the vocal organs, but if we return to our stage-by-stage consideration of speech production, we can consider next initiation: that is, the process of setting an airstream in motion. For most of speech we use a pulmonic egressive airstream, in other words a stream of air flowing out of the lungs. It must be remembered, though, that other airstreams are possible (those used for ejectives, implosives and clicks, see Ball 1993). Nevertheless, most experimental phonetic work in this area has been concerned with measuring pulmonic airflow (both ingressive as in breathing in, and egressive as in breathing out or in speech), and also sometimes in comparing oral and nasal airflow. This area of experimental study is called 'aerometry', and considerable developments have been made in the instrumentation used here.

Aerometry systems normally utilize an airtight mask which fits over the mouth and nose. The mask contains a number of sensors that measure air pressure and airflow. Normally it is possible to measure both ingressive and egressive airflow, and to distinguish oral from nasal flow. As phoneticians usually wish to compare airflow measurements with specific aspects of speech, the mask will contain a microphone to record what the subject is saying. Aerometry systems are today linked to computers, and software allows us to display flow patterns in conjunction with the speech signal, so we can see with what sounds airflow increases and decreases, and to spot the correlation, for example, between increased nasal airflow and the production of nasal consonants and nasalized sounds.

Phonation

Following initiation, we can consider phonation: that is, vocal fold activity in the larynx during speech. There are several different ways in which we can investigate vocal fold activity. One of these involves working out from the acoustic record of speech the fundamental frequency of the speaker's voice (that is to say the frequency of vocal fold vibration). We shall return to acoustic methods of analysis in Chapter 6. In terms of articulatory instrumentation we can use either direct observation of vocal fold action, or indirect measurement. A variety of direct observation apparatus is available, but most of this involves the use of an endoscope. An endoscope is a long thin tube, either rigid or flexible, through which the relevant laryngeal activity can be seen. Rigid endoscopes have to be inserted orally (and very carefully!), whereas a flexible endoscope can be inserted via the nasal cavity and into the pharynx. Clearly, only the second type allows for anything resembling natural speech: if a rigid endoscope is used, only sustained vowels can be investigated. To enable the investigator to see the vibrations of the vocal folds, stroboscopic light (i.e. rapidly flashing on and off) can be fed down fibre optics in the endoscope, and using the same technology, video recording can be made from the endoscope.

However, such direct measuring techniques are invasive, in that the insertion of the endoscope is bound to affect the naturalness of the speech. Many investigators, therefore, have preferred the use of the electrolaryngograph (ELG), also known as the electroglottograph (EGG). This technique allows us to work out the patterns and frequencies of vocal fold vibration by measuring electric current flowing across the folds. Electrodes are carefully placed on the neck of the subject so as to be either side of the larynx. A tiny electric current is passed along the system, so when the vocal folds are together current can pass through the larynx and complete a circuit. When the folds are parted, this circuit is interrupted. Computer technology can then use this information to provide detailed patterns of vocal fold activity, from which we can calculate changes in pitch, as well as patterns of phonation. Many ELG systems also contain software to allow the user to undertake a series of acoustic analyses to plot alongside the vocal fold data. We return to such analyses in Chapter 6.

Velic action

Before we can consider the articulation of individual speech sounds, we must remember that a major division of such sounds concerns the use or otherwise of the nasal cavity as well as, or instead of, the oral cavity. Nasal resonance can be added to otherwise oral sounds (for example to produce the nasal vowels of languages like French and Portuguese); and of course the nasal stop sounds, such as [m] and [n], use the nasal resonator only.

It is often important in clinical phonetics to be able to ascertain how much nasal airflow is being used by a speaker, and what percentage of the overall airflow at any one time is oral and what is nasal. Although it is possible to use acoustic measurements in this area (see Chapter 6), it is more direct to use adaptations of the aerometry procedures referred to above. *Nasometry* is the term often used to describe this approach, and various proprietary devices are available that attempt to measure the egressive oral and nasal airflows of speakers, with computer software doing analyses such as calculating percentage oral/nasal flow. The drawback with many of the cheaper devices is that separation of the two airflows may be through the use of a simple metal plate, held against the face, rather than through an airtight mask, and the measurements may be made through the use of microphones to detect the noise of the airflow, rather than the more accurate airflow sensors.

Articulation – EPG

To examine articulation itself, two distinct approaches can be taken: devices using artificial palates, and imaging techniques. The most common artificial palate-based technique is *electropalatography* (EPG; also termed electropalatometry). This requires the subject to be fitted with a very thin plastic artificial palate on which are fixed a large number of tiny electrodes (62–96, depending on the system used). The electrodes are fired when there is contact between them and the tongue. Wires leading from the artificial palate out of the mouth are connected to a computer, which scans the patterns of fired and unfired electrodes many times a second (e.g. 100 times a second for the Reading EPG3 system) and so can display in real time the ever-altering patterns of tongue–palate contact during speech.

It has to be borne in mind, however, that this system can investigate only articulations that involve a contact or near contact between the tongue and the hard palate, and the front edge of the soft palate. Therefore, places of articulation such as bilabial and labiodental at one extreme, and uvular, pharyngeal and glottal at the other are excluded. Also, manners of articulation such as vowels and semi-vowels may show some patterns of contact for the side rims of the tongue (if they are for example high front vowels or semi-vowels), but little else. Also, because EPG is measuring what happens at the palate, it cannot be as clear when it comes to the tongue shape. We cannot be sure, for example, in the production of the approximant [ɹ] of many English accents, whether the tongue tip is slightly retroflexed, or whether it is bunched. The contact patterns may help us with an educated guess, but cannot guarantee our analysis.

Further, differences between oral and nasal sounds, and voiced and unvoiced (or aspirated and unaspirated) cannot be shown in EPG, and these clearly need the use of instrumentation referred to earlier. Finally, we should note that palate shapes differ from speaker to speaker, and so comparing results of EPG across subjects must be undertaken with care.

To surmount the problem of the inability of EPG to show tongue patterns for vowels, researchers are still working on a system which would use an artificial palate to transmit and detect light. The idea is that tiny fibre optics would carry the light, and that the time taken from the light to leave the transmitter, 'bounce' off the surface of the tongue, and then reach the receiver would be interpreted by a computer and displayed as movements of the tongue surface in the vertical dimension.

However, this system, like EPG, is still limited in terms of place of articulation, though it may well be able to provide more information on tongue shape than can EPG. If we want further information on articulation, then we must use imaging techniques.

Articulation – imaging techniques

Imaging techniques are methods whereby the investigator obtains an image of the interior of the vocal tract, or some part of it, to enable them to measure position and in some cases movement of the vocal organs. The image may either be directly of the structures of the vocal tract itself, or may consist of the tracks of special metal pellets attached to important points of the vocal tract (such as the tip of the tongue). We can therefore term the first category *structural imaging*, and the second *tracking*.

Among the structural imaging types are radiography, ultrasound and magnetic resonance imaging (MRI). Tracking techniques include X-ray microbeam, and electromagnetic articulography (EMA). We shall now look at these briefly in turn.

Radiography

Radiography is the oldest of the imaging techniques used for investigating speech. Within a few years of the discovery of X-rays in 1895, radiographic images of the upper vocal tract were taken by phoneticians. X-rays, like light, heat and radio waves, belong to the electromagnetic spectrum of rays, and are at the low-frequency end of the spectrum. They are useful in the analysis of speech articulation because of three important properties. First, X-rays penetrate material which absorbs and reflects light. Second, the rays are absorbed to greater or lesser degrees, depending on the density of the material: the denser the material, the greater the absorption of the X-rays, and vice versa. Therefore, if X-rays are recorded on photographic plates or on cine or video, different densities will be decipherable. Finally, X-rays travel in straight lines, and are not easily refracted or reflected.

Many X-ray techniques have been developed, including still, cine and video pictures; more specialist techniques also exist, including panoramic radiography, kymography, tomography, xeroradiography and X-ray microbeams (discussed in more detail later).

One of the most popular speech disorders on which X-rays have been used for analysis is the *craniofacial* disorder. An example of such a disorder is *cleft palate*, and X-ray has been used in the past as either a descriptive tool for it (e.g. Shprintzen *et al* 1980), or for the purposes of diagnosis (e.g. Bowman and Shanks 1978). X-ray has also been used to compare disordered speakers with normal speakers (e.g. Glaser *et al* 1979). The postoperative assessment of patients is another common area in which X-ray is used, in order to monitor their progress after the operation. This was used by Enany (1981), who measured the effects of primary osteoplasy in unilateral cleft lip and palate patients.

It is, however, the very property that makes radiation therapy effective for treating disease that has limited its use in speech research: it can damage or kill living cells and, for this reason, access to X-ray equipment is strictly monitored.

Ultrasound

Ultrasound measurements give information about the tongue and the larynx during articulation. This is because ultrasonic pulses (sounds with frequencies of 2–20 MHz) reflect off physical structures, such as the larynx and the tongue; by measuring the time it takes for the pulses to be reflected back to the transmitter, distances moved by the articulators can also be derived. The ultrasound transducer is held against the skin underneath the chin, and the sound waves pass into the tongue. Once the waves reach the airspace in the oral cavity, they are reflected back to the transducer. Images of the tongue or larynx are then reconstructed from the reflected echoes, and displayed on either an oscillograph or a computer screen.

The instrumentation necessary to carry out an ultrasound investigation comprises an ultrasound generator, an amplifier, an A/D converter and an oscillograph or computer. For tongue measurements, the transducer is placed under the chin of the subject, along the midline of the mandible; in a study of vocal fold vibrations (Kaneko *et al* 1981) the transducer was placed on the thyroid lamina.

Ultrasound investigations have dealt primarily with tongue movement and shape, which is important in the analysis of grooved and slit fricatives, and in examining tongue shape in vowels.

Magnetic resonance imaging

The magnetic resonance imaging technique (MRI) is used mainly in medical circles to obtain details about the inside of the human body. In recent years, the technique has also been applied to studies on speech.

In an MRI investigation, a large magnetic field is applied to biological tissue, e.g. the vocal tract. This tissue contains many hydrogen atoms, which have a nuclear magnetic resonance signal, and which therefore become aligned parallel to the magnetic field. Radio wave signals are then sent to the part of the body under investigation by an antenna, signals are emitted and sent back to a receiver. These signals are converted, by means of a processor unit, into an image. More details of the technical specifications of MRI instrumentation may be found in Westbrook and Kaut (1993). One drawback of the technique is that currently, only static images can be obtained because of the time required to produce the image. One study (Westbrook 1994) states that it takes 6 seconds; another, carried out a year later (Foldvik *et al* 1995) quotes 1 second. Instrumentation is, however, rapidly developing, and in the future it may be possible to produce images more quickly.

Studies using MRI images have concerned vocal tract measurement (Rokkaku 1986), pharynx shape during the production of vowels (Baer *et al* 1987, Lakshiminarayanan, Lee and McCutcheon 1991, Greenwood, Goodyear and Martin 1992), nasals (Dang *et al* 1993) and fricatives (Narayanan, Alwan and Haer 1995). The images have also been used to construct models of the vocal tract, which were then used to synthesize four vowels (Baer *et al* 1991). As yet, there have been few studies using MRI on disordered speech, although it is expected that this will change in the near future.

X-ray microbeam

The X-ray microbeam is a tracking technique which uses very small doses of X-rays (controlled by computer) to record the movement of pellets attached to the tongue. The technique is non-invasive, holds little risk for the subject, and has been used to investigate both normal and disordered speech.

A study by Hirose *et al* (1978) used X-ray microbeam to examine articulatory movement in dysarthric speakers. These speakers had different types of dysarthria: one had ataxic dysarthria of cerebellar origin, the other had amyotrophic lateral sclerosis. X-ray microbeam was employed to look for differences in articulatory movement which would distingush different types of dysarthria, as well as to detect the central problems of speech production in such patients. It is therefore a useful technique for making clinical diagnoses, and for searching for possible remedies for speech disorders. The technique has also been used to study articulation in apraxic speakers (Itoh *et al* 1980) and in patients with Parkinson's disease (Hirose *et al* 1981). The major disadvantage of this useful technique is its expense.

Electromagnetic articulography

EMA is also a tracking system, which provides information on speech kinematics, and again is useful in analysing articulatory movements in both normal and disordered speakers. Three commercially produced EMA systems are currently available: The Carstens Electromagnetic Articulograph AG 100 (Schönle *et al* 1987, Tuller, Shao and Kelso 1990), the Electromagnetic Midsagittal Articulometer EMMA (Perkell *et al* 1992) and the Movetrack from Sweden (Branderud 1985). These systems comprise a lightweight helmet, small connector coils which are placed in and on the speaker's mouth and a unit for connection to a computer.

The transmitter coil generates an electromagnetic field, the strength of which decreases the further the coil is placed from the transmitter. A receiving coil is placed parallel to the transmitter, and induces an alternating low voltage. Transmitter coils with different frequencies are used, and the distance between the transmitter and receiver can be calculated from the strength of the voltages induced in the receiver.

Further reading

Readers interested in more details on any of these techniques may consult relevant chapters in Ball and Code (1997) and Lass (1996). Illustrations of some of these approaches, and their application to speech-language pathology, are given in the following chapter.

CHAPTER 5

Articulatory Analysis of Disordered Speech

In the previous chapter we saw a range of instruments that can be applied to the study of speech articulation. Naturally, these can be used to investigate disordered as well as normal speech. However, in this chapter we shall concentrate on just three techniques: electropalatography, magnetic resonance imaging (MRI) and nasometry.

Electropalatography

This technique is especially useful for investigating (and treating) articulation disorders: in this case we mean specifically problems in correct tongue–palate placement and control. Electropalatography (EPG) has been used with a wide variety of speech disorders: cleft palate, developmental articulation disorders, disfluency and acquired articulation problems (such as dysarthria and apraxia of speech). In this section we shall look at four studies, two reported in a special EPG issue of the journal *Clinical Linguistics and Phonetics*; one dealing with apraxia of speech, and one with cleft palate. The first of these used EPG primarily as an investigative technique, while the second employed it also in therapy. The third study investigates Pierre Robin sequence, and the final one looks at covert contrasts in the acquisition of phonology.

Edwards and Miller (1989) report the case of a 58-year-old male subject with a left posterior temporo-parietal infarct. He was investigated with EPG on various tasks one year after a cerebrovascular attack. The speech error investigations were centred around three tasks: single word production, single word repetition and spontaneous sentence production (each sentence containing one item from the single word list). Interestingly, the different tasks produced different numbers of errors, with the repetition task proving to be motorically most difficult for the subject. The items were all transcribed and checked against the EPG printout. The authors found that although they had auditorily detected most of the errors, there were some that were only discovered after the EPG frames had been studied. This shows that impressionistic transcription cannot always tell us what is going on with the speech production process simply because some articulatory gestures may be 'hidden' (or overlaid) by others, and because the same (or very similar) acoustic patterns may be produced by different configurations of the vocal organs.[1]

Among the articulations that were found to be difficult to transcribe were target /tʃɪə/ transcribed as [kɪə]. Although the EPG record clearly shows that the patient was able to produce an alveolar-postalveolar contact pattern at the beginning of the relevant segment, a velar stricture was formed during the production of the sound, and was released after the anterior contacts. This led to the percept of a velar sound, but it is clear from the EPG evidence that this was not a simple case of velar substitution. The subject was also required to undertake various non-linguistic oral tasks: such as repeating [tʌtʌ] and [tʌkʌ] patterns. The EPG evidence supported the view that although the subject was aware of the target he was aiming at, he had difficulty in controlling the movements and the timing involved in these tasks.

Gibbon and Hardcastle (1989) investigated a 13-year-old boy, whose hard palate had been repaired only two years earlier (though lip and soft palate repair had taken place much earlier). Impressionistic analysis of the subject's speech led to the conclusion that alveolar plosives and nasals had been backed to the velar position, and alveolar grooved fricatives sounded palatal with accompanying posterior nasal friction. Other sounds appeared normal, though in connected speech there seemed to be an increase in the posterior nasal friction.

An EPG analysis was also undertaken to test these initial findings. We saw above that auditory impressions do not always correspond strictly to the tongue–palate contact patterns recorded by EPG. However, in this case, the EPG printouts supported the impressionistic transcription. Figure 5.1 shows the subject's (above) and a normal speaker's (below) contact patterns for /n/ and for /t/ in the word 'knot', and Figure 5.2 shows patterns for the /ʃ/ in 'shop'. Although the palato-alveolar fricatives had been heard as normal, the EPG printout in Figure 5.2 shows that they, like the alveolar fricatives (not illustrated here), had a palatal realization. Figure 5.1 bears out the perceived alveolar to velar changes.

---

[1] This can be exemplified in normal speech in English. The approximant /r/ of most accents of English can be produced with two different tongue configurations, known as the retroflex-r and the bunched-r (see Ball and Rahilly 1999 for illustrations), yet both sound the same.

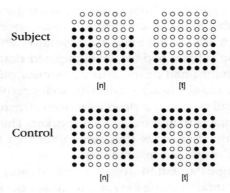

Figure 5.1. The subject's (above) and a normal speaker's (below) contact patterns for /n/ and for /t/ in the word 'knot'. (Adapted from Gibbon and Hardcastle 1989).

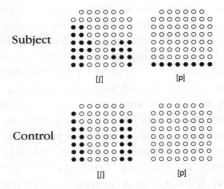

Figure 5.2. The subject's (above) and a normal speaker's (below) contact patterns for the /ʃ/ and /p/ in 'shop'. (Adapted from Gibbon and Hardcastle 1989).

However, the EPG also showed up something that had not been detected auditorily. The subject consistently used a velar contact as well as a labial one when producing /b, p, m, f/. This double articulation was only detected through EPG, showing the value of articulatory instrumentation in the clinic.

Three main aims were established for the subject in therapy:

• to eliminate double articulation with bilabials
• to establish anterior contacts for alveolar plosives and nasals
• to establish more anterior and closer grooved productions of the alveolar and palato-alveolar fricatives

EPG was used with the patient, who was old enough to have the technique explained and to be able to use it to monitor his own speech. The therapy lasted for 14 weeks in 1-hour sessions. After therapy, EPG investigations demonstrated that the subject had totally eliminated double articulation with the labial consonants; had nearly normal anterior placement for the alveolar plosives and nasal (though still with some atypical palatal and posterior contacts); and /s, z/ had a clearer grooved structure, though still with more palatal contacts than for a normal speaker. The palato-alveolar fricative showed minimal changes (but remember that this sound had sounded 'normal' in the initial transcription).

The subject's long-established atypical articulation patterns were generally successfully treated using EPG as a feedback device as well as an assessment tool. Final impressionistic transcriptions suggested only slight unusual articulations with the alveolar fricatives, with other sounds recorded as normal.

Howard (1998) describes a case of Pierre Robin sequence. This is an unusual condition associated traditionally with three main symptoms: micrognathia (small lower jaw), cleft palate and upper airway obstruction (often caused by the tongue falling back into the pharynx). Howard's subject in this study had not received glossopexy (suturing of the tongue tip to the lower lip to avoid the airway obstruction), but had had a tracheostomy. His cleft palate had been repaired at the age of 2. He had undergone speech therapy (concentrating on language abilities rather than articulation) since the age of 3, and at 6 years old his speech was impressionistically described. Howard (1998) notes that at this time the subject was able to signal the oral/nasal contrast well, but that phonatory activity was abnormal leading to a hoarse, aperiodic voice quality. Nevertheless, phonological voicing contrast was usually maintained.

The subject did have, however, considerable difficulties in manipulating the fine tongue control needed to produce the full range of place and manner contrasts in the consonant system. The broad groupings of plosive, fricative and approximant were normally successfully achieved, but the distinction between plosives, affricates and fricatives was not. Lateral approximants, also, were missing from his system. It is difficult to be sure, of course, whether these sounds were not established phonologically, or whether the motor control and co-ordination problems referred to made it difficult for him to realize a contrast that had, indeed, been internalized.

In terms of place contrasts, the subject achieved bilabial and velar targets well, but was much less successful with alveolar and post-alveolar ones. For example, target alveolar fricatives were realized as bilabial, palatal and velar. It was felt that these place of articulation problems were one of the major causes of unintelligibility in the subject's speech.

This subject was reassessed at the age of 13: this time the impressionistic description was backed up with EPG. Although therapy had
continued, this had still not been aimed at phonology or articulation.
Therefore, the subject still presented with many of the problems
described above. In particular, auditory impressions suggested that alveolars and post-alveolars were being consistently realized further back in the
vocal tract as palatals or velars.

Using EPG data, Howard was able to look at the variability in the
subject's articulations, and also at how similar different alveolar targets
were. Interestingly, the stops /t/ and /n/ differed from the fricative /s/. The
patterns for /s/ and for /ʃ/ were very similar and showed a minimal amount
of variability. The articulation of these sounds involved tongue–palate
contact at the borders of the palatal-velar area. On the other hand the
stops showed a great amount of variation: for /t/, for example, the subject
consistently made a closure, but the location and width of this closure
varied, both between words and between repetitions of the same word. As
with /n/, though, the locations were generally alveolar, post-alveolar or
occasionally a little further back. Finally, the subject's attempts at /l/ can be
considered. These were judged to be atypical, and the EPG evidence bore
this out. No alveolar contact was achieved, and contact was restricted to
the two margins of the palate (as Howard points out, the opposite of what
is required).

This study does not describe any future therapy plans, but it would be
interesting to see whether EPG could be used in a remediation scheme, as
well as being an assessment tool.

Gibbon (1990) looks at what she terms here as 'subphonemic cues', or
elsewhere as 'covert contrasts' in both normal and disordered phonological acquisition. We have already noted in some of the studies referred
to above the fact that EPG can reveal that two articulatory gestures that
produce the same auditory impression may result from different arrange-
ments of the vocal organs. Thus, we may have contrasts produced by the
speaker, which are lost to the listener: 'covert contrasts'. In her 1990
paper, Gibbon was one of the first to look at these. What makes this case
study particularly interesting is that the two subjects were sisters (MB aged
4;10, and VB aged 6;2). Both had an array of simplifying processes, but
whereas MB was recorded as backing alveolars to the velar position, this
was not a process noted for VB. EPG recordings of both sisters were
undertaken using both real and nonsense words. The 1990 article concen-
trates only on the alveolar–velar contrast, in particular using the nonsense
pair [da:] – [ga:], and compares the production of the two sisters with that
of a normal speaker.

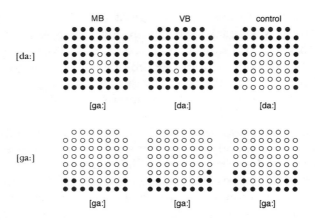

Figure 5.3. Frames of maximal contact for [da:] – [ga:] for MB, VB and control subject. (Adapted from Gibbon 1990).

In Figures 5.3 we show the point of maximum contact for the target syllables for MB, VB and the control subject. It can be seen from this figure that all three subjects produce very similar patterns for [ga:], but that for [da:] the two sisters have a very different pattern from the control. This patterns shows contacts across both the alveolar and velar regions for MB and VB, whereas the control has contacts restricted to the alveolar section. How is it, then, that only MB was recorded as backing alveolars to velars? If we look at Figure 5.4 we find the answer. This figure shows the tongue–palate contact patterns at the point of release of the stops. Again, the [ga:] tokens are all very similar. For [da:], however, whereas VB releases her velar contacts before her alveolar ones (thereby producing a release burst that is acoustically similar to that of the control subject), MB releases her alveolar contacts first and velar ones last, thereby producing a release burst that sounds like that of [g].

This study demonstrates two things: first, that covert contrasts can exist in a speaker's repertoire though inaudible to the listener. MB clearly has a different pattern of articulatory behaviour when producing target [d] and [g], even though they both sound the same. Her problem, then, is not phonological: she does not have a problem in separating these two sounds at the organizational level. Her problem is one of motor implementation and co-ordination. The second finding is the converse: what may sound correct (as in VB's productions of target [d]), may not always result from an articulatory configuration and sequence we would expect to find as the most economical, and that we do find in typical speakers.

Of course, VB's results do not affect her ability to signal phonological contrasts, and so have little implication for therapy. MB's, on the other

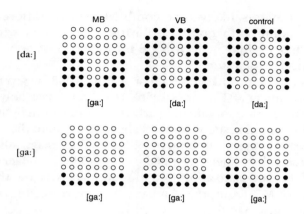

Figure 5.4. Frames just prior to stop release for [da:] – [ga:] for MB, VB and control subject. (Adapted from Gibbon 1990).

hand, are important. EPG shows us where the problem lies in this case: phonologically based approaches to intervention stressing the importance of contrastivity would be wasted with this subject. MB demonstrates she knows the sounds contrast. What is needed is therapy aimed at the articulatory level – perhaps using EPG itself as a feedback tool.

Magnetic resonance imaging[2]

Imaging techniques for the investigation of speech have in recent years become more sophisticated and wide-ranging, to some extent in response to the decline in popularity of radiographic approaches. Furthermore, the application of these new developments to the study of disordered speech has become more popular. In this section we aim to describe magnetic resonance imaging (MRI) (see Ball and Gröne 1997).We describe the kind of images these systems can produce, and the relative strengths and weaknesses of the technique, particularly when applied to a variety of speech disorders in research and clinical applications.

MRI (or nuclear MRI) is a non-invasive imaging technique giving three-dimensional views of biological tissue with good resolution compared to many other approaches (particularly of the soft tissue of the vocal tract). Its main drawback currently is temporal, in that, due to the time required to obtain an image, static images only are possible (though recent developments towards a more dynamic system can produce images very frequently). It is only recently that MRI has been applied to speech (see

---

[2] This section is a simplified version of a section appearing in Ball, Gracco and Stone (2001).

below), but it seems likely that combinations of different imaging techniques – some with good resolution, and others with dynamic temporal abilities – may well provide information of great interest to speech scientists in the future.

Nuclear magnetic resonance was first seen in 1945 by groups of scientists at Stanford and at MIT (Morris 1986). However, it was only in the early 1970s that MRI was developed, and early studies in the analysis of (among other areas) biological tissue were published. Since then, there has been a dramatic increase in the application of MRI to medical diagnosis and, as just noted, more recently to speech. Rokkaku *et al* (1986) and Baer *et al* (1987) were some of the earliest to apply MRI to speech analysis, but the continual improvement of MRI equipment means that more recent publications show clearer images than those in this early work.

The majority of MRI studies on speech have concentrated on examining the vocal tract, and comparing MRI results with those obtained from other methods (such as the acoustic record or radiography). Rokkaku *et al* (1986) were interested in vocal tract measurement, and Baer *et al* (1987) looked at pharynx shape during the production of the vowels /i/ and /ɑ/ in two subjects. The results of this latter study were checked with radiographic data from the same subject, and it appeared that the dimensions obtained from the two methods did not fully agree: the MRI results were significantly larger than those from the radiographic study. Various sources of error were suggested to account for this discrepancy (including body posture), but it did not prove possible to explain them unambiguously.

Baer *et al* (1991) built on this first study by adding data for the vowels /æ/ and /u/, together with axial pharyngeal images of the vowels /ɪ, ɛ, ɔ, ʊ, ʌ/. In this study also, the authors used the MRI images to build models of the vocal tract which they then used to resynthesize the four vowels /i, æ, ɑ, u/. The real and synthesized versions were played to a panel of naive listeners who had to identify which vowel they heard. Although the real data were recognized correctly more often than the synthesized data, the differences were slight. Other recent MRI studies of vowel production can be found in Lakshminarayanan, Lee and McCutcheon (1991), and Greenwood, Goodyear and Martin (1992).

Investigation of errors in MRI data was one of the main aspects of Moore (1992). The author used various analysis procedures to calculate vocal tract volumes from the MRI scans, and to see how these fitted in with well-established acoustic transmission theory. Five subjects were used in the investigation, which looked at a limited set of both vowel and consonant articulations. Interestingly, one of the subjects had a slight articulatory disorder, in that sibilants were produced with noticeable lateral distortion; this appears to be one of the first MRI studies to include any account of disordered speech.

Moore's results clearly demonstrate the lateral articulation of /s/ with the subject noted above. However, more interestingly, the article describes sources of error in analysing images and ways of correcting these. Finally, the resulting vocal tract volumes obtained from the study, when applied to acoustic resonance theory, accurately predict the acoustic make-up of the vowels studied. Moore believes, therefore, that MRI can be used effectively in studies of speech production. Figure 5.5 illustrates one of the images obtained during this study, and demonstrates tongue position for the English vowel /u/.

Other studies mainly concerned with modelling the vocal tract, or aspects of it, include Foldvik *et al* (1993), and Yang and Kasuya (1994); Foldvik *et al* (1995) compare MRI with ultrasound. Studies are also beginning to appear that examine specific classes of speech sounds. We have noted above various vowel studies; there have now been studies on nasals (Dang, Honda and Suzuki 1993), and fricatives (Narayanan, Alwan and Haer 1995). Demolin *et al* (1997) examined coarticulation in connected speech via MRI: an area of great potential for future studies.

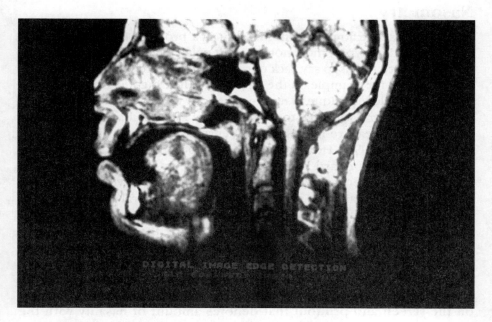

Figure 5.5. MRI image for the vowel /u/. (Courtesy of C. Moore).

Masaki *et al* (1999) describe a study using an external trigger to coordinate a series of repeated MRI scans with the subjects' beginning of the test utterance. Subjects repeated test utterances 128 times, from which 35 frames were constructed into the equivalent of an MRI film. Selected frames were compared with those obtained from a static study where the subject sustained a particular segment for 1 second: long enough for the scan to take place. Comparisons demonstrated that in the sustained mode, tongue–palate contact for /k/ and tongue alveolar ridge contact for /t/ appeared wider than in the dynamic mode. Sustaining such articulations would appear, then, to distort the normal contact patterns due to the need to maintain a closure over time. The dynamic frames also clearly displayed interesting coarticulatory effects between alveolar and velar consonants and a following /a/ vowel that would not easily be seen in a sustained mode.

Clearly, we are only at the beginning of research using MRI. We can confidently predict that studies of disordered speech using this approach will be reported in the literature with increasing frequency. It may well be that MRI will continue to be used with other dynamic systems for the time being, but if image acquisition times can be improved still further, it could become one of the dominant techniques in speech imaging.

Nasometry

Excessive nasal airflow, or hypernasality, is a problem encountered in a variety of patient types, most notably cleft palate. Less common, perhaps, is hyponasality, that is to say, lack of nasal airflow when it is required. This can be found, for example, in the language of hearing-impaired speakers. Clearly, a simple technique to measure nasality that could be used also for therapy would be a useful tool. Aerometry systems have traditionally been used to measure ingressive and egressive airflows in speech (see Zajac and Yates 1997). However, these are expensive pieces of equipment and not straightforward to use. In recent years simpler (though less reliable) instruments have been designed. These have been termed nasometry devices and use microphones to measure oral and nasal egressive airflow, and rather than requiring an airtight mask over the face, generally employ a simple metal plate to divide the nasal microphone from the oral one (see Ball 1993). The Kay Elemetrics Nasometer was the first of such instruments to gain widespread recognition; however, more recently Awan and colleagues have developed a new instrument, NasalView, which, among other things, allows the user to line up the trace on the screen and printout that denotes amount of nasality with the acoustic waveform so that it becomes easy to see at which point in an utterance a particular change in nasalance occurs. Awan *et al* (1999) describe the application of this piece of equipment to the analysis of nasalance in patients who had undergone secondary osteoplasty for cleft palate. The analysis presented in this article was based on over 140 patients: 45 with perceived normal nasal resonance, 38 with mild hypernasality, 33 with moderate and 27 with severe. Numbers of hyponasal patients were too small to be included. The purpose of the study was to see how well this particular instrument could distinguish between the groups of patients already established by perceptual means. Subjects were tested on sentences rather than single words.

Awan *et al* were interested in looking at how well the NasalView instrument diffferentiated between normal and different types of hypernasal speakers. Two measures were drawn up: *sensitivity* – that is, whether subjects were included in a group who should be, and *specificity* – that is, whether subjects were excluded from a group who should be. The overall results indicated that, when comparing normals to moderate and severe hypernasal subjects, the authors obtained a sensitivity rating of 90% and a specificity rating of 73%. When comparing normals to just severely hypernasal patients the scores were 91% and 89% respectively. It will clearly be interesting to watch the future refinement of this instrument, as a tool for both assessment and therapy with hypernasal subjects.

Coventry, Clibbens and Cooper (1998) describe what they term a 'new speech aid', specifically designed with therapeutic feedback in mind. This instrument (the PSL: postable speech laboratory) combines acoustic information (in the form of the speech waveform), electrolaryngraphic data in the form of a larynx wave reflecting vocal fold activity, and airflow traces from both the mouth and the nose. The article describes some of the evaluative procedures undertaken to test the PSL, and also presents a brief case study of a 16-year-old patient who used PSL as a feedback tool. For our purposes here, however, it will suffice to demonstrate the possibilities of the PSL by reproducing one of the printouts. Figure 5.6 shows the printout for a normal speaker uttering the word 'mean'. The audio waveform shows the difference between the nasal segments and the intervening vowel, and the larynx wave shows that voicing continues throughout the utterance. As we should expect, the oral and nasal airflows traces are almost mirror images: as the nasal airflow increases during the nasal consonants, the oral airflow decreases. However, these two traces also demonstrate that the vocal segment has coarticulatory nasalization, and that this is strongest in anticipation of the following nasal consonant, but dies away swiftly following the first one. The PSL demonstrates the usefulness of combining a range of instrumental approaches to phonetics, and we return to this topic in Chapter 10.

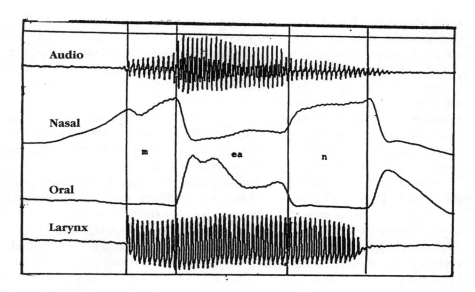

Figure 5.6. Printout of 'mean' from PSL. (From Coventry, Clibbens and Cooper 1998; courtesy of the authors).

Further reading

A range of chapters in both Ball and Code (1997) and Lass (1996) will add depth to some of the discussion here.

CHAPTER 6

Acoustic Instrumentation

In order to understand how acoustic instrumentation works, we first need to grasp some basic acoustic properties and terms. Speech acoustics is the study of the transmission of speech from the speaker to the hearer through the air. In other words, acoustic phonetics looks at speech once it has left the organs of articulation and before it operates on the organs of hearing. In studying this area of phonetics, we need to know about how sound actually travels through the air, and the various parameters we can measure as it does this, in order to classify speech sounds according to their acoustic make-up. In the first section of this chapter, therefore, we shall examine the notion of sound waves, frequency and duration, amplitude and intensity, and resonance. Following on from discussing these terms, we shall look at how instrumentation has developed to measure these acoustic features, and what this can tell us about speech.

Sound waves

All sound results from a vibration of some sort, which in turn depends on a source of energy to generate it. An example often cited is that of a symphony orchestra, in which the players generate vibrations by carrying out various actions, such as blowing or hitting. The vibrations produced by these actions result in sound waves.

Sound waves are produced by the displacement of air molecules, which occurs when a sound is made. This displacement is caused by variations in air pressure, which – if the sound in question is a speech sound – are generated by movements of the speaker's vocal organs. These waves travel through some medium (usually air), propagating outwards from their source in a manner similar to ripples on a pond, until they reach the eardrum of the hearer and cause it to vibrate.

There are many different kinds of sound, and thus many different kinds of sound wave. The simplest type of sound wave is known as a *sinusoidal*, or more usually, a *sine* wave. This is the type of wave produced, for example, by a tuning fork when struck. The prongs of the fork vibrate, moving from side to side of their rest position, and when this displacement is plotted against time, a sine wave is produced. As Figure 6.1 shows, the line of displacement curves up from the axis (representing rest position), and then curves down, meeting the axis again and continuing downwards to show displacement in the opposite direction. When it curves upwards to meet the axis for the second time, we say that one *cycle* has been completed. Repetition of these cycles continues, though not indefinitely, as in practice, energy is lost due to friction and air resistance. This process is known as *damping*.

As stated above, the sine wave is the very simplest type of sound wave. Speech sounds, on the other hand, have complex waveforms, often made up of a series of simple sound waves. Each sound has its own characteristic waveform, which is determined by the position and actions of the vocal organs during the production of the sound. Complex waves can be categorized as being *periodic* or *aperiodic*. Periodic sounds have a regularly repeated pattern of vibration; aperiodic sounds have random vibrations which are not regularly repeated. Vowels are an example of a class of sound which has a periodic vibration, while voiceless fricatives have aperiodic vibrations. Figure 6.2 shows an illustration of a vowel waveform, and Figure 6.3 of a voiceless fricative waveform.

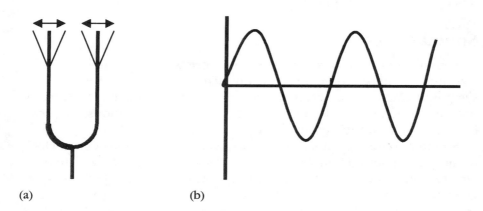

(a)   (b)

Figure 6.1. Sine wave: (a) tuning fork; (b) sine wave, showing displacement on the vertical axis and time on the horizontal axis.

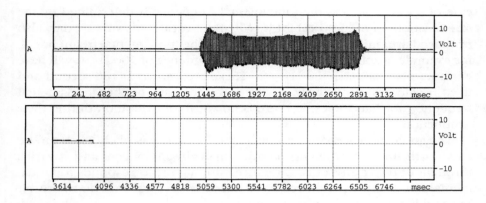

Figure 6.2. Vowel waveform [i].

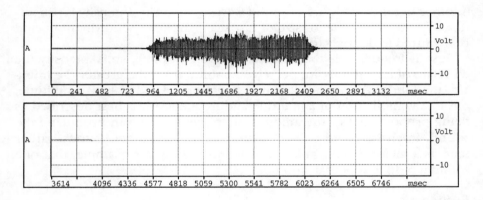

Figure 6.3. Voiceless fricative waveform [ʃ].

Frequency

One important aspect of the sound wave is its frequency. This is a technical term which refers to the number of cycles, i.e. the number of complete repetitions of movement from the starting position through the displacement positions and back to the starting position, occurring every second. The unit of measurement of frequency is the Hertz, usually abbreviated to Hz, so if a sound wave has 150 complete cycles in a second, we say that the frequency of the sound is 150 Hz.

Periodic sounds have a fundamental frequency, which is provided by the lowest frequency of the sine waves which make up the sound; in the case of speech sounds, the fundamental frequency is determined by the rate of vibration of the vocal folds. When the vocal folds vibrate, they also produce harmonics, which are multiples of the fundamental frequency. If, for example, a sound has a fundamental frequency of 100 Hz, it will have harmonics of 200 Hz, 300 Hz, etc. These are known as the second and third harmonics respectively. Voiceless sounds have neither fundamental frequency nor harmonics, as there is no vocal fold vibration during their production.

The auditory correlate of fundamental frequency is pitch. Pitch can be used both linguistically and paralinguistically in speech, and it varies throughout the course of an utterance. Although it corresponds to fundamental frequency, equal increases or decreases in frequency do not result in equal increases or decreases in pitch.

Intensity

Another significant feature of sound waves is intensity. Intensity is proportional to the amplitude, or size of displacement in a sound vibration, and is measured in decibels (dB).

Just as frequency is the acoustic correlate of pitch, so is intensity the correlate of how loudly we perceive a sound; thus, the greater the intensity, the louder the sound. It is not, however, related only to amplitude, but to a combination of amplitude and frequency; it is best described as being proportional to the amount of energy involved in producing the sound. Intensity is normally measured relative to other sounds, rather than as a measurement in itself, so we would say, for example, that one sound is 5 dB louder than another.

Resonance

The setting in motion of one system by the vibrations of another is known as *resonance*, an important phenomenon in explaining the quality of a given sound. The way in which vibrations from one system can be transmitted through another can be illustrated using a spring mass (see Figure 6.4).

If periodic vibrations are applied to the system by vibrating the anchoring point, these are input vibrations, and the consequent vibrations at the bottom of the spring mass are output vibrations. The spring mass is a mechanical system, which has a natural, or *resonant* frequency, and this determines how it responds to input vibrations. If, for example, the frequency of the input vibration is much lower than the resonant frequency, the amplitude of the output vibrations will be low. The same applies if the input vibration frequency is much higher. The output vibration amplitude will be at its maximum when the input vibration frequency is equal to the resonant frequency. The energy of the input vibration is thus transmitted selectively by the resonant system.

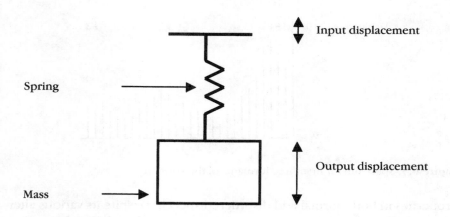

Figure 6.4. Resonance.

In speech, the vocal tract acts as the driven system, and it is the vibration of the vocal folds which sets in motion the air in the vocal cavity. Since the driving force is a complex tone, containing more than one frequency, the driven system (vocal tract) will select those that are at, or nearest to, its resonant frequency and increase their amplitude. These peaks of amplitude are known as *formants,* and these are the resonant frequencies of the vocal tract for the sounds in question. The vocal tract can alter its shape, which means that formants occur at different frequencies for different sounds and, in fact, it is the formant structure which determines the quality of a sound. The formant structure of a sound can be illustrated diagrammatically in a sound spectrum.

The spectrum shows frequency on the horizontal axis against intensity on the vertical. They are drawn from a single moment during a speech sound, and display the first three formants in a voiced sound. Figure 6.5 shows a spectrum for the vowel sound [i].

Acoustic analysis

The spectrograph

Since the 1940s, the sound spectrograph has been the instrument most commonly used in investigating the acoustic properties of speech. As is the case with all technological instruments, the spectrograph has substantially changed and developed since its invention, and in recent years has become even more sophisticated and efficient with the advent and development of computerization. This allows for the automatic analysis of digitized sound signals, and the spectrograph is used to display various acoustic

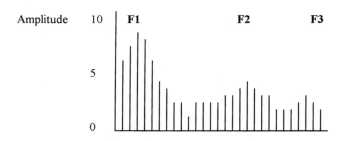

Figure 6.5. Spectrum for first three formants of the vowel [i].

properties in both normal and disordered speech. Despite its various alterations, the essence of the spectrograph has remained unchanged.

The spectrograph produces a diagram called the *spectrogram*, which displays the spectral analysis of speech sounds, plotting frequency against time. In order to achieve this visual representation, the spectrograph analyses the speech sound into its component frequencies, and passes those frequencies which fall within a certain range, without reducing their energy. This range is called the *bandwidth* of the filter, and those frequencies that fall outside it have their frequencies reduced to a very low level. This type of selection process, whereby certain frequencies are selected and passed without a reduction in their intensity, while others have their intensity reduced, is carried out by the *bandpass filter*, which is a type of resonant system. A spectrograph may, for example, have a filter bandwidth of 45 Hz, and thus may pass frequencies within the 45–90 Hz range. This means that any frequencies falling within that range are selected and their intensities displayed; whereas any falling outside of that range will have their amplitudes greatly reduced. The darkness of the display corresponds to the intensity of the sound, so frequencies with greater intensities will register as darker than those with lesser intensities. The formants of a sound are therefore displayed as dark horizontal bars.

Spectrograms may be either *wide-band* or *narrow-band*. Narrow-band spectrograms respond to frequencies within a narrow band, e.g. 45 Hz, whereas wide-band spectrograms respond to those within a much broader band, e.g. 300 Hz. The choice of one type over another depends on whether the speech analyst is more interested in the frequency or in the time component. This is because one of the characteristics of a system with a narrow bandwidth is that there is very little damping. This means that it takes some time (20 ms for a 45 Hz bandwidth) before new information can be dealt with, and that any new information occurring within that gap is lost. A system with a broader bandwidth, on the other hand, has a much quicker time resolution (3 ms for 300 Hz) although it does not provide such precise frequency information. Speech analysts are normally more concerned with the formant structure of sounds over time than they are with precise frequency details, and for this reason the wide-band spectrogram is the more commonly used.

Acoustic measurements

Formants

As stated above, spectrography can be used to make various acoustic measurements. One important measurement in speech is that of the formant structure and formant frequencies of voiced sounds. All voiced sounds have a fundamental frequency and harmonics, some of which are emphasized, depending on the resonant qualities of the vocal tract. These emphasized harmonics are the formants, and every voiced sound has a characteristic formant structure. Although most sounds have several formants, speech analysts are usually concerned mainly with the first and second formants, and indeed describe vowel sounds in normal speech in terms of the relationship between the first and second formants (often called F1 and F2). The formant structure of vowels is discussed in more detail below. The frequencies at which formants occur are influenced by the height of the tongue, the anterior–posterior positioning of the tongue and the degree of rounding or protrusion of the lips.

An analysis of formant structure can also made in the examination of disordered speech. Past studies have, for example, investigated whether or not F1 and F2 values show more vowel centralization in the speech of non-stutterers than that of stutterers (Prosek *et al* 1987), and have found that F2 values may be missing or unmeasurable in stutterers (Yaruss and Conture 1993). In a study carried out on cerebral palsy sufferers, it was found that formant relationship and transition is important in influencing the intelligibility of their speech (Ansel and Kent 1992).

Segmental duration

The spectrograph is also used to examine segmental duration in both normal and disordered speech. When measuring stop consonants, voice onset time (VOT) is used; this is the time between the release of the articulators involved in the stop and the beginning of voicing, and is measured in milliseconds. This can be done very easily and accurately on a computer, as cursors can be placed at either end of the segment in question, and their values displayed automatically. Vowel duration is another frequently made measurement, which again may be easily made using the spectrograph. Past studies have shown that tense vowels are longer in duration than lax vowels, that close vowels are longer in duration than open vowels, and that vowels that precede a voiced consonant are longer in duration than those that precede a voiceless consonant.

Segmental duration is also important in the study of disordered speech. Research has found, for example, that VOT is longer in stutterers than in non-stutterers, as is consonant and phrase duration (Healey and Ramig 1986). Throneburg and Yairi (1994), on the other hand, found that there was no significant difference between the duration of spoken units in stutterers and non-stutterers, but that stutterers had shorter silent intervals than non-stutterers. Apraxic subjects were shown to have markedly longer vowel durations than normal-speaking subjects (Collins, Rosenbek and Wertz 1983) and non-fluent aphasic speakers also had longer vowel durations in certain conditions (Duffy and Gawle 1984).

The following section examines the acoustic characteristics of specific classes of sounds, which can be displayed on the spectrograph.

Acoustic characteristics of vowels

The precise acoustic make-up of vowels, or indeed any sound, varies both between speakers, and within the speech of the same speaker. There are, however, acoustic features which sounds have in common, regardless of inter- and intra-speaker variations.

Vowels are, in almost all known languages, voiced, which means that they have a formant structure showing peaks of energy. Each vowel has a formant structure which indicates vowel height, tongue advancement and lip shape. The first formant (F1) corresponds to tongue height: close vowels have lower F1 values, and open vowels have higher F1 values. Cardinal vowels 1–4 would therefore display a progressive increase in the frequency value of the first formant, whereas cardinals 5–8 would have a progressive decrease in F1 values. F2 usually reflects the front–back position of the tongue, with front vowels having higher F2 values than back vowels. Lip-rounding is indicated by a lowering of all of the formant values.

Vowel spectrograms also have a voicing bar, which is a band of energy, indicating the fundamental frequency (F0) value, and normally lies between 100 and 200 Hz. Voicing is also reflected by the vertical striations that can be seen running throughout the sound.

Acoustic characteristics of diphthongs

Diphthongs involve a movement of the tongue from the position required for one vowel sound to that required for another. This results in a change in the formant structure in the course of the spectrogram, so that it displays a combination of the characteristic patterns for both components of the diphthong.

Acoustic characteristics of plosives

Plosives involve a closure of the articulators, an accumulation of air pressure behind them, followed by a release of the articulators. These stages are reflected on the spectrogram: the closure phase is marked by a period of silence, with no energy markings, apart from a voice bar in the case of voiced plosives, and the release phase is marked by a burst of widely spread noise energy, whose peaks occur at different frequencies according to their place of articulation. In the case of alveolar plosives, for example, the second formant is usually between 1700 and 1800 Hz. It may be, of course, that the stop is not released, in which case it is marked only by a break on the spectrogram.

Acoustic characteristics of fricatives

In the production of fricative consonants, there is not a complete stoppage of air, as there is in plosives. Instead, the air is forced through a narrow channel between two articulators. This results in noise energy occurring at very high frequencies, which again are located on the spectrogram according to their place of articulation. The labiodental [f], for example, usually has its energy peak between 6000 and 8000 Hz.

Acoustic characteristics of affricates

An affricate is a combination of a stop and a fricative, and the acoustic characteristics of both types of sound can be seen on the spectrographic display. This means that there is a break for the stop, which, instead of being followed by a burst of noise corresponding to the plosive release, is followed by high frequency noise, corresponding to the fricative component of the affricate.

Acoustic characteristics of liquids

Liquids contrast with plosives and fricatives, in that they involve no obstruction of the airstream. These sounds are thus acoustically similar to vowels, in that they have a voicing bar and formants. This section focuses on the acoustic characteristics of the English liquids, [l] and [ɹ]. When examined on the spectrogram in inter-vocalic position, the liquids are seen to be shorter than the surrounding vowels. The retroflexion which is found in most varieties of the English [ɹ], is displayed on the spectrogram, where the third formant lowers and then rises during the production of the sound. The principal acoustic characteristic of [l] is the abrupt transitions of the first and second formants.

Acoustic characteristics of nasals

In the articulation of nasal consonants, the velum is raised to block off the oral tract, resulting in the expulsion of air only through the nasal tract. Nasal sounds therefore have a lower intensity than oral sounds, and this is reflected on the spectrogram by a lighter trace. Another characteristic is that when compared to a neighbouring vowel, the first formant is lower than that of the vowel. This is a result of an antiresonance introduced by the nasal sound, and is normally located in the 800–2000 Hz range.

Pitch

We saw above that pitch is the acoustic correlate of the frequency of vibration of the vocal folds (the fundamental frequency). Pitch – or intonation – may be used for many purposes in speech: it may be used semantically, so that the meaning of a phrase changes depending on the pitch pattern employed by the speaker. For example, the phrase *John's here* implies a statement, and in Southern British English, would be pronounced with falling pitch, whereas the phrase *John's here?* is a question, and is likely to be pronounced with rising pitch. Pitch may also have a syntactic function, in that it breaks up passages of speech into smaller linguistic units. It can also have an emotive or affective function, and can express excitement, nervousness, sadness, boredom, and many other emotions. Pitch patterns, like segmental patterns, vary according to accent and dialect.

Phoneticians and phonologists often differ in opinion as to the most suitable transcription system for intonation patterns, and may also differ in their opinions as to what the various pitch patterns occurring in a particular dialect may mean. Most researchers, however, share the belief that the domain of intonation is the phrase, and that each phrase has a particularly important word, in terms of its informative value, attached to which is a particular pitch movement, e.g. a *rise*, a *fall*, or a *fall-rise*.

Electrolaryngography

Electrolaryngography is a technique used to monitor vocal fold activity, and can thus be used to examine intonation patterns. It does so by means of two electrodes placed on the skin of the neck on each side of the thyroid cartilage, and is therefore a non-invasive technique. A weak electric current is passed through the larynx from one electrode to the other, and the effects of the varying impedance of the vibrating vocal cords on the current gives information about the vocal cord activity. The resulting display (called the Fx waveform) may be shown on an oscilloscope screen or, more usually nowadays, on a computer screen.

Electrolaryngography can, of course, provide other information about the larynx, other than the pitch patterns that are produced by vocal fold vibration. The Lx trace, for example, gives information as to the type of voice, e.g. it may be creak or whisper, and also displays information about the voiced/voiceless state of the glottis. This area is discussed in more detail later.

Visi-Pitch

A narrow-band spectrogram may also be used to analyse intonation patterns, but this is difficult to read, and is no longer the most popular method of measurement. A number of commercially produced instruments have been introduced in recent years, which give an automatic reading of the pitch curve. An example of such a product is the Visi-Pitch instrumentation, produced by Kay Elemetrics. Recent versions of the Visi-Pitch can interface with computers, and can make a statistical analysis of the results found, e.g. the highest and lowest fundamental frequency values. Instruments such as this are useful in the remediation of pitch disorders, as the patient may see on the screen the pitch track which they are to attempt to reproduce, and may compare their own production with that of the therapist to monitor progress.

Connected speech

The acoustic descriptions of the consonant and vowel sounds given in this chapter have concerned discrete speech sounds. However, in practice, speech is not normally produced in terms of isolated sounds, but consists of sounds that overlap, and which are influenced by their surrounding segments. This can be seen in a spectrographic analysis of some formant structures. For example, in the case of a vowel following a bilabial stop (/p/ or /b/), the second formant moves upwards.

Voice quality

Another aspect of connected speech is voice quality types. The acoustic features of the various phonation types can be examined both spectrographically and by using the electrolaryngograph. Modal voice – that most often found in normal speech – may be compared with other voice quality types, some of which are found in other languages, and some of which are found in disordered speech. Creaky voice, for example, is found in disordered speech, and is characterized by a low frequency vibration of the vocal folds. This can be recognized on the spectrogram by the very clear vertical striations, which are more spaced out than those that would be found in modal voice. The laryngograph waveform display shows a regular, slow vibration of the vocal folds.

Whisper is another phonation type that may be found in disordered speech. In this voice type, there is no vibration of the vocal folds; however, the vocal tract is still capable of producing the resonances necessary for comprehensible speech. The formant structure for vowels will therefore still be present, although the voicing bar will not. Since there is no vocal fold vibration, the electrolaryngograph is of no use in the analysis of this phonation type. It should not be confused with whispery voice (or murmur), which does have voicing as well as a discernible formant structure.

Supraglottal voice quality types, e.g. palatalized and nasalized, can also be analysed on the spectrogram. Palatalized voice involves the raising of the tongue towards the hard palate, and the spectrographic display will therefore have characteristics similar to an [i] vowel, i.e. the second formant is likely to be higher than expected. In velarized voice, on the other hand, the second formant is likely to be lower than normal, as it would be in the vowel [u].

Further reading

Farmer (1997) and contributions to Lass (1996) may be consulted. Denes and Pinson (1973), Fry (1979), Kent and Read (1992) and Johnson (1997), among many others, also have good introductions to acoustic phonetics.

CHAPTER 7

Acoustic Analysis of Disordered Speech

The principles and practice of acoustic analysis described in Chapter 6 can be applied to a very wide range of speech disorders. Nevertheless, for this approach to be of use, the clinical phonetician must not only be able to understand the spectrogram or other acoustic detail produced via analysis, they must also be able to detect differences between the acoustic data of the disordered speaker and that of a normal and know when such differences are important.

First in this chapter we are going to examine a study where the use of acoustic analysis was crucial to attempts by clinical phoneticians to transcribe the speech of a severely disfluent speaker. This was a particularly problematic case, as the tape recording used was old, had been recorded in noisy conditions, and was recorded on basic equipment. Nevertheless, as we shall see, acoustic analysis was able to overcome these drawbacks in many respects. Second, we shall take a brief look at how acoustic analysis can aid in the investigation of disordered vowel systems. Our final example will demonstrate how we can use acoustic analysis to examine segment durations in a speaker with apraxia of speech.

The disfluency study[1]

The subject was a young adult male stutterer (Mr S), aged 24 at the time of recording. He presented with severe stuttering behaviours, present since early childhood. His accent was Belfast English (see Milroy 1981).

In spontaneous speech, he used excessive struggle behaviours and facial grimacing in an effort to control his speech, which was characterized

---

[1] An earlier version of this study was presented in Ball and Local (1996).

by part-word repetitions of plosives and fricatives, and severe blocking on word-initial sounds. He had particular difficulty with initiating voicing at sentence boundaries, due to an intermittent ingressive gasp of air, or intrusive nasal snort. Ingressive airflow was also found in other situations (see transcript below).

Although lacking in self-confidence, he persisted with the target sound or word, often up to 10 s, until he managed to produce it (e.g. 'towns' in the transcript). However, excessive facial and body tension distracted the listener further from the message to be communicated. Further details of this subject are given in Ball *et al* (1994).

The recording was made at least 10 years before the authors undertook this analysis. It was made on a cassette recorder using a built-in microphone, and the recording took place in a clinic room of a speech therapy facility which lacked any kind of sound-proofing. Indeed, noises from the outside corridor are sometimes audible, and at the end of the passage transcribed, one can hear someone knocking on the clinic room door. Such conditions are, of course, contrary to almost all the criteria normally laid down for recording material for phonetic analysis. However, as noted above, in clinical phonetics, ideal conditions often cannot be found.

A passage was chosen for transcription where the subject was reading from a prepared text. This had the advantage that we knew what the target utterances were. Furthermore, as this task was quite stressful for the subject, it meant that we should be likely to find a good number of disfluencies of various types to deal with. The transcribers (the authors) found normal measures of inter-transcriber reliability difficult to calculate, as several parts of the passage could not be dealt with at all because the speech was so quiet, or caused considerable uncertainty because of the rapidity of the reiterations.

The passage read was as follows:

The World Cup Finals of 1982 are held in Spain this year. They will involve the top nations of the world in a tournament lasting over four weeks held at fourteen different centres in Spain. All of the first round games will be in the provincial towns, with the semi-finals and final held in Barcelona and Madrid.

The first attempt at impressionistic transcription using both extIPA and VoQS conventions and symbols together with standard IPA symbols produced the following incomplete attempt:

1.
[ð\ð:ǝ̰ {V̰ ǝ\ǝ\ǝ V̰} 'hw̥ɔːld 'kʌp 'f\faməlz ǝv 'naɪntɪn eǝti {↓p 'tŭ p ↓} ,ɑː 'h\held

ɪn sːp\sːp\ʰeǝn 'ðɪs jɔɹ (3 secs) ǫ̈ːe wɪl ɪnv\'y̰ːɔlv ðǝ ((untranscribed 4 sylls)) fŋ \

{f fŋ \ fŋ f }\ţŏp̚ 'neʃǝnz ǝv ðǝ 'wɔɹld ɪn' ǫ̈ ((untranscribed 3 sylls))\ ţ̣ʉɪnǝmǝnt

'lastɪn ,ouvǝɹ 'fɔɹ 'wiks (..) 'ḥeld ǝ\ ʔat 'f\fɔɹtɪn (...) ((reiteration x3?))\ 'dɪfɹǝnt

'sen{↓tǝɹz̰↓} ɪn 'speǝn (3 secs) ǫ̈ (.) 'ɔl ǝv ðǝ f\f 'ɔl ǝv ðǝ 'fɔɹ̣t 'ɹaʉnd 'geǝmz

wɪl bi (..) wɪl bi (.) ɪn ðǝ (.) w̰ǫ̈ː p\pɹǝv\'vɪnʃǝl ((untranscribed 6 sylls?)) fŋ \ fŋ

\ {↓tãũnz↓} wɪð ðǝ ((reiteration x3?)){↓emi 'faməlz↓} and 'f\famǝl 'held ɪn (.)

((*)) bɑɹsǝ{p 'loʊnǝ and 'mǝdɹɪdp }]

* knock on the door
N.B. Predictable vowel length not marked. Predictable consonant quality (e.g. aspiration) not marked on fluent items.

Before we go further, we should at this point explain some of the transcriptions in (1) above for those not familiar with extIPA and VoQS (see Chapter 3). Curly braces (i.e. {}) enclose stretches of speech for which specific prosodic information is encoded. This may be ingressive airstream – marked with ↓ – or a voice quality, such as creaky voice (i.e. V̰), or loudness, where $_p$ and $_{pp}$ mark quiet and extra quiet respectively.

Reiteration is marked with the backslash \, and this occurs frequently in this example. Reiteration is defined by extIPA as being rapid repetitions of segments or syllables; where pauses occur between repetitions, or elsewhere, they are marked by the period within braces: (.). Longer pauses are marked with extra periods up to three; but it is recommended that pauses of more than a couple of seconds should be noted in figures, e.g. (3 secs). Information on background noise or incomprehensibility is put in double braces.

There is one segmental symbol in the transcription above not found in the IPA: [fŋ]. This is an extIPA symbol for the velopharyngeal fricative (also termed the 'nasal' or 'velopharyngeal snort'), and was commonly used by this subject during struggle behaviour occuring in prolonged disfluent passages. There is also one extIPA diacritic: [̬] which denotes strong articulation (particularly noticeable after a reiterated section).

At this stage, it became clear that we should need to investigate the acoustic record instrumentally to deal with the unclear passages. Although it might be argued that what one cannot hear should not be transcribed, there were clearly some passages where the problem was the speed of reiteration and others where a quiet voice combined with bad tape quality interfered with the transcription process. We would argue this is different from features that are impossible to hear in normal circumstances with non-speech-impaired subjects. Furthermore, it is also valuable to record aspects of the speech production process that can be discovered only through instrumental analysis if we wish to extend our models of this area.

The tape of the entire passage was spectrographically analysed by the Signalyze 3.11 package, operating on a Macintosh Powermac 6100/60 computer. Particular attention was paid to the five parts of the passage where the initial impressionistic transcription had been uncertain. These sections were looked at with as high a time resolution as possible, although some of the surrounding parts of the passage were also included in this examination to aid in the interpretation of the resultant wide-band spectrograms.

The five spectrograms are reproduced below as Figures 7.1–7.5, and each shows the initial transcription assigned to the passage as a result of the examination of the acoustic record. Further information (such as degree of loudness, or voice quality) was added later, as this information was not always obvious from the spectrograms, because of the large amount of background markings resulting from the background noise of the original tape recording.

The first uncertain section followed immediately after the words 'will involve the', and it became clear from examining the spectrogram shown in Figure 7.1, that we had here an example of reiterated attempts at the initial [t] of 'top', followed by the velopharyngeal snorts that were

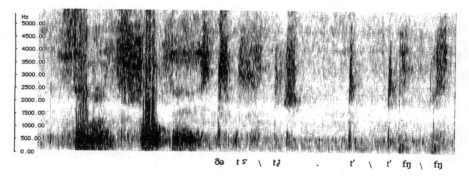

Figure 7.1. Spectrogram of problem passage 1.

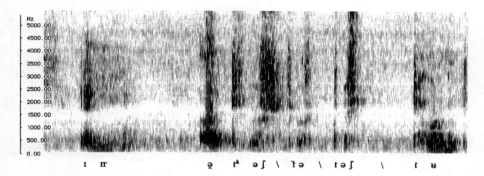

Figure 7.2. Spectrogram of problem passage 2.

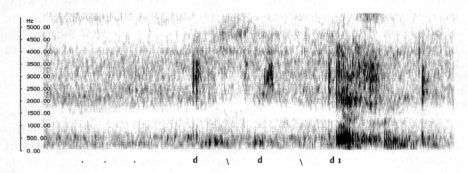

Figure 7.3. Spectrogram of problem passage 3.

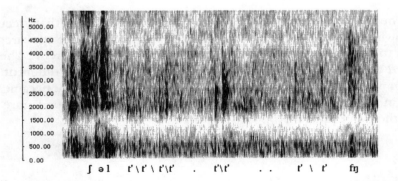

Figure 7.4. Spectrogram of problem passage 4.

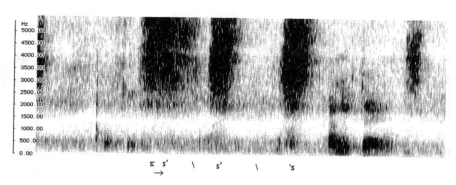

Figure 7.5. Spectrogram of problem passage 5.

transcribed in (1) above. Initially, it had seemed that these reiterations differed in quality, and we were able to confirm this impression on the spectrogram, where different types of friction were visible after the first two plosive releases. Putting this information together with our impressions of the sound quality, we propose a transcription for this section as follows:

2. [tˢˌ\tᴶ (.){p t'\t' p}]

The second section examined consisted of a series of reiterations in the phrase 'in a . . . tournament'. Again, we see a problem with initial [t], and again there appears to be the inclusion of some fricative elements following the release of the stop (see Figure 7.2). Our proposed transcription for this section is:

3. [{pp tʰ'ə∫\tʰə\tə∫ pp}\]

The third portion we looked at was a reiteration that occurred following the pause after the words 'at fourteen . . .', and appeared this time to be a reiteration of the initial [d] of the word 'different'. This was heard as being probably three repetitions before [d] of 'different', but when we looked closely at the spectrogram of this section, it became clear that in fact only two plosive release lines could be seen (see Figure 7.3), and the transcription proposed is thus:

4. [{pp V̰ d\d V̰ pp}\]

The voice quality and loudness characteristics in this transcription were added by the transcribers to reflect their impressions of this section. The background noise shown on the spectrogram unfortunately did not allow voice quality information to be displayed clearly.

The fourth section was a long series of reiterations, again connected with an attempt at an initial [t]; in this case of the word 'towns' following the word 'provincial'. In this instance, the question facing us was the number of reiterations, as opposed to issues of sound quality, as much of the section was spoken with a very quiet voice. The spectrogram shown in Figure 7.4 was able to show us clearly that there were eight (as opposed to our initial estimate of six) repetitions before the velopharyngeal snorts that were transcribed into the initial attempt in (1) above. We show our transcription as:

5.   [{p t'\t' p} \ {pp t'\t' pp} (.) t'\t' (..)   {pp t'\t' pp}]

The final section consisted of a reiteration at the beginning of the word 'semi-final'. Our initial estimate was that there were three repetitions of [s] before the [s] of 'semi-', but we were not certain as to the exact quality of each example. The spectrogram shown in Figure 7.5 suggests that there are only two examples of [s] before 'semi-', with the first of these an extra-long example. However, it is clear when listening to the first example, that the [s] after being held for a while is closed as an ejective [s'], whereas the second example is an ejective [s'] only. To show this we have used the extIPA convention of the arrow beneath two symbols that represents sliding articulation: in this case sliding from a normal [s] to an ejective [s'].
We show the final transcription as follows:

6.   [sːs'\s'\'s]
         →

This exercise has demonstrated how useful the acoustic record can be in resolving problematic aspects of phonetic transcription. It must be remembered, however, that acoustic analysis is only one instrumental technique that can be brought to bear on difficult material. Recent developments in articulatory measurement (for example through the use of electropalatography, or electrolaryngography) can help resolve transcriptional uncertainties as well; often these may be more helpful than relying on spectrography. However, many of these techniques cannot be used with taped material, as they require the subject to be connected to the instrumentation. In the case of our sample, therefore, acoustic analysis was the only realistic option open to us.

If we put all these transcriptions together, we can show the entire passage as below:

7.

[ð\ð:ə̯ {V̥ ə\ə\ə V̥} 'hwɔ̯ɪld 'kʌp 'f\faməlz əv 'naɪntin eəti {↓p 'tŭ p ↓} ,ɑɹ 'h\held

ɪn s:p\'s:p\ʰeᵊn 'ðɪs jəɹ (3 secs) ɵ̯̈ :e wɪl ɪnv\'v̥:ɔlv ðə tˢˑ\ʈɹ (.) {p t'\ʈ' p} fɲ \ {f fɲ

\ fɲ f }\ʈ ɒ̯p' 'neʃənz əv ðə 'wɔɹld ɪnˑ ə̯ {pp tʰəʃ\ʈʰə\təʃ pp}\ ʈ ʉɪnəmənt 'lastɪn

,oʊvəɹ 'fɔɹ 'wiks (..) 'held ə\ ʔat 'f\fɔɹtin (...) {pp V̥ d\d V̥ pp} \ 'dɪfɹənt

'sen{↓tɜɹz↓} ɪn 'speᵊn (3 secs) ə̯ (.) 'ɔl əv ðə f\f 'ɔl əv ðə 'fəɹʂt 'ɹaʉnd 'geᵊmz

wɪl bi (..) wɪl bi (.) ɪn ðə (.) w̥ə̯: p\pɹəv\'vɪnʃəl {p t'\ʈ' p̯} \ {pp t'\ʈ' pp} (.)

t'\ʈ' (..)   {pp t'\ʈ' pp} fɲ \ fɲ \ {↓tãũnz↓} wɪð ðə s:s̯'\s'\'s{↓emi 'faməlz↓} and

'f\faməl 'held ɪn (.) ((*)) bɑɹsə{p 'loʊnə and 'mədɹɪdp }]

* knock on the door
N.B. Predictable vowel length not marked. Predictable consonant quality (e.g. aspiration) not marked on fluent items.

Disordered vowel systems

There has been a marked increase in interest in disordered vowel systems in the last 10 years or so; see Ball and Gibbon (2001 forthcoming) for a full review of this area. This work has demonstrated that it is not true that phonological disorders are restricted to consonant systems and that vowels can therefore be ignored in profiles or tests of phonology. However, whereas the transcription of consonants (even consonants from outside the phonological system of the target language) can be learnt comparatively easily, the transcription of vowels has proved problematic. As Ladefoged (1967) showed, even trained phoneticians can experience difficulty in the transcription of vowel sounds markedly different from those found in their own language. It is true that the cardinal vowel system (see Chapter 1), if learnt properly, should help clinical phoneticians to describe even the most unusual vowel (unusual in terms of the target system, of course). However, not all speech pathology courses do introduce this system or, if they do, do not devote enough time to it. Also, individual students do differ in how well they learn the system: Ladefoged's study showed that although phoneticians trained in the cardinal vowel system did outperform those who were not in vowel identification, even they encountered problems.

We therefore need an alternative to impressionistic transcription when it comes to vowel description; or at least, something to augment our transcriptions. Acoustic analysis is ideally suited to this task. As noted in Chapter 6, vowels can be identified by the first three formants (in many cases the first two will suffice). Modern acoustic analysis equipment can provide various ways of accessing information on the formant structure of vocalic segments. Not all these ways will produce identical results (different ways of measuring acoustic events will often produce somewhat differing data), but as long as one is consistent in the measure being taken, then the segments measured will all be in the same relation to one another.

Naturally, if the disordered vowel system being investigated is simply an example of phonological neutralization, then recourse to acoustic analysis may not be needed. By phonological neutralization we mean that certain phonological units that are contrasted in the target form may be merged into just one of these units in the client's speech. We can illustrate this by considering the three vowels of English *beat, bit* and *bet*, normally transcribed /bit, bɪt, bɛt/. If these three vowels are merged into, for example, the /i/ vowel, then we have neutralization. The resultant system will be smaller than the target system, but the vowels will be straightforward to transcribe as the reduced system consists of units that are phonetically the same as a subset of the target system. The problem arises if the client's system is partly or completely phonetically different from the target. This may co-occur with neutralization, of course. We could think of a variant of our previous example, whereby the three mid and high front vowels merged into a vowel not found in the target system (e.g. [œ] or [ɵ]).

Particularly problematic for English transcribers are front rounded vowels, back unrounded vowels, and central rounded vowels. Although these may well be unusual realizations of vowels in English, it is still necessary to be able to deal with them should they occur. To this end, we show in Figures 7.6–7.9 diagrams of the formant structures of some of these vowels ([y, ø, ɤ, ɯ]) spoken by an adult female with no speech disorder. (See Chapter 2 for a description of the vowel symbols used in this section.) Linear predictive coding (LPC) analysis was undertaken at the mid point of each vowel, and values for F1, F2 and F3 recorded. These values are shown in Table 7.1, and can be compared to values for female speakers for normal English vowels given in Table 7.2 (derived from Peterson and Barney 1952).

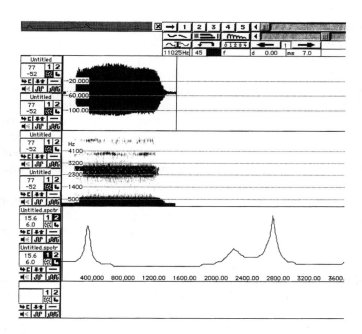

Figure 7.6. Spectrogram and LPC of the vowel [y] (Prepared by Dr Joan Rahilly).

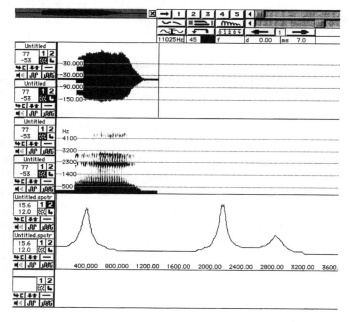

Figure 7.7. Spectrogram and LPC of the vowel [ø] (Prepared by Dr Joan Rahilly).

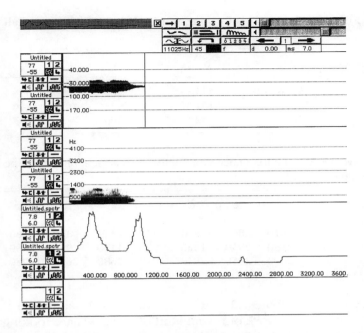

Figure 7.8. Spectrogram and LPC of the vowel [ɤ] (Prepared by Dr Joan Rahilly).

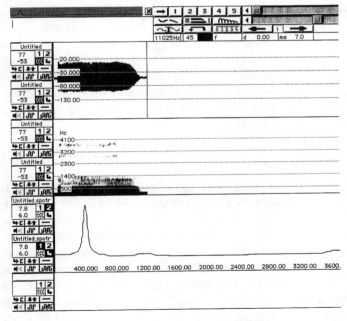

Figure 7.9. Spectrogram and LPC of the vowel [ɯ] (Prepared by Dr Joan Rahilly).

Table 7.1. Formant frequencies for four non-English vowels for an adult female speaker

Formant (Hz)	y	ø	ɤ	ɯ
F1	344	414	367	398
F2	2233	2171	992	1140
F3	2725	2842	2303	3607

Table 7.2. Average formant frequencies for English vowels for adult female speakers of American English

	i	ɪ	ɛ	æ	ɑ	ɔ	ʊ	u	ʌ	ɚ
F1	310	430	610	860	850	590	470	370	760	500
F2	2790	2480	2330	2050	1220	920	1160	950	1400	1640
F3	3310	3070	2990	2850	2810	2710	2680	2670	2780	1960

We can see from Table 7.2 that values of F1 and F2, and to a lesser extent F3, can help us work out what kind of vowel we are looking at. F1 values help us with tongue height: high vowels have a low F1 whereas low vowels have a high value. F2 helps us with tongue advancement: front vowels have higher F2 values than back vowels. Lip-rounding has the effect of lowering energy levels throughout the formants compared to non-lip rounded vowels. With this aid to reading acoustic analyses of vowels, the clinical phonetician should be able to identify even those vowels least like any within the target system. However, vowels may differ from the target in ways other than formant structure: durational differences may also be found (with consonants as well, of course). We turn our attention to duration in the following section.

Segment duration

In this section we report on a study undertaken by Code and Ball (1982). In this investigation the authors examined the production of English fricatives in a Broca's aphasic patient, and it transpired that duration measurements were of primary importance in the description of this subject's speech: and duration can be accurately measured only through acoustic analysis.

Before we examine this case, it is worth remembering that fricatives in English are distinguished by a series of phonetic features: place of articulation, voicing, duration of frication and duration of preceding vowel. The members of the four fricatives pairs /f, v/, /θ, ð/, /s, z/, and /ʃ, ʒ/ are distinguished as follows:

- The first in each case is voiceless (lacks vocal fold vibration), the second usually has some voicing (fully voiced intervocalically, partially voiced in word initial and final positions).
- The first in each case has a longer frication duration than the second.
- Vowel length before the first in each case is reduced as compared to that before the second.

In this account we term the first member of each pair *fortis,* and the second *lenis.*

The subject in this case clearly had difficulty in integrating the voicing component with the production of fricatives, although voicing was not a problem in the production of sonorants (such as nasal consonants or vowels). The subject was a 63-year-old right-handed female Broca's patient, three years post-onset. The patient exhibited no signs of dysarthria. An age and sex matched control speaker was included in the investigation.

A list of 17 pairs of words was produced that were minimal pairs or near minimal pairs of voiced and voiceless fricatives, with the fricatives in initial (e.g. 'fine–vine'), medial (e.g. 'proofing–proving') and final position (e.g. 'pence–pens'). The experimental and control subjects were recorded reading this set of words, and the recorded data were later subjected to spectrographic analysis. The first part of the analysis concentrated on the evidence for voicing in the spectrographic record. The experimental subject had no voicing at any point during either the fortis or lenis fricatives. On the other hand, the control showed patterns of voicing during the lenis fricatives as would be expected for English (see above). This suggested that the experimental subject was merging the fortis–lenis contrast in these fricatives.

However, when durations were examined, a different picture emerged. Two durational measurements were taken: duration of the vowel preceding the fricative (clearly this applied only to medial and final fricatives), and the duration of the frication itself (i.e. the period of turbulent airflow). The mean values for these durations are given in Table 7.3.

These figures show that, despite the loss of ability to produce vocal fold vibrations at the same time as fricative consonants, the experimental subject is controlling one of the other main acoustic cues for the fortis–lenis distinction well: the length of preceding vowels. The figures for both subjects in this regard are remarkably close. The third acoustic cue (duration of frication) is, however, somewhat more problematic. The experimental subject does make a difference in the duration of frication between fortis and lenis pairs of fricatives, but this difference is much less than that made by the control (47 ms compared to 73 ms). Furthermore, the durations of the fortis and lenis fricatives is greatly increased in the

Table 7.3. Vowel and fricative durations

	Experimental subject		Control subject	
	Vowel duration	Fricative duration	Vowel duration	Fricative duration
Fortis	176 ms	223 ms	159 ms	176 ms
Lenis	247 ms	175 ms	232 ms	104 ms
Difference	71 ms	48 ms	73 ms	72 ms

speech of the experimental subject as compared to that of the control (by around 50–75 ms). Figure 7.10 shows a spectrogram of the English words 'safe' and 'save' said by a normal speaker. Each word on the spectrogram consists of a central dark area surrounded by paler areas. The dark areas represent the vowels, the lighter areas the fricatives. The time scale in milliseconds at the base of the spectrogram can be used to measure the durations of these components.

It would appear that the loss of one of the cues to the fortis–lenis distinction in fricatives (voice) has led the experimental subject to compensate by overemphasizing another. That this is the frication duration cue (rather than the vowel length one) makes sense, as this is a cue embedded within the consonant itself. Such findings also strongly support that notion that apraxia of speech is not a phonological impairment (otherwise the lenis fricatives would simply have been merged with the fortis), but rather a phonetic level one. In particular, a phonetic

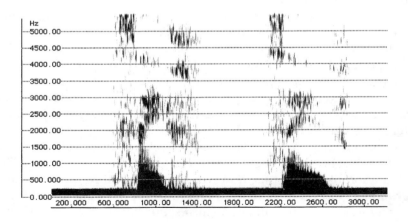

Figure 7.10. Spectrogram of the English words 'safe' and 'save'.

implementation impairment. We say this as it is clear the speaker can produce all the relevant phonetic features (voice, friction), and can manipulate duration. What she was unable to do was to co-ordinate all these features simultaneously.

Without access to spectrographic analysis, studies like this one are impossible. Fine degrees of duration difference, presence versus absence of slight amount of voicing, and so on, are simply not analysable accurately through transcription alone. Acoustic analysis systems are simply essential in the clinical phonetics laboratory.

Further reading

Farmer (1997) describes acoustic analysis for clinical phoneticians. Contributors to Lass (1996) describe in detail a range of experimental techniques.

CHAPTER 8

Auditory and Perceptual Instrumentation

In describing the instrumentation commonly used in the field of auditory phonetics, it is necessary to describe the mechanisms involved in the hearing, the perception and the comprehension of speech. Hearing relates to the physiological operations of the different parts of the ear, and this part of the auditory system is known as the *peripheral auditory system.* Perception and comprehension involve the neural activity which decodes the speech signal into meaningful units and relates them to semantic concepts, so that it can be understood. This aspect is known as the *internal auditory system.* This chapter describes these auditory systems, describes the various types and causes of hearing loss, looks at the important aspect of *feedback,* and discusses some auditory techniques and their instrumentation.

The auditory system

Once a sound wave travels through air and reaches the ear, it is transmitted through the outer ear, the middle ear and the inner ear. This section describes this process.

The part of the ear that can be seen outside of the body is known as the *pinna* or *auricle.* At this point, the sound wave enters the ear canal (or the *external auditory meatus*), which acts as a resonator, and has a resonant frequency of between 3000 and 4000 Hz, although this varies according to the individual. It will therefore amplify sound waves with frequencies close to its own resonant frequency. The ear canal ends at the eardrum, or *tympanum*, which is where the middle ear begins. The eardrum membrane has an area of approximately 0.75 cm² and a thickness of approximately 0.01 cm.

The middle ear is an air-filled cavity, which contains three bones (or *auditory ossicles*) attached to its walls by ligaments. One of these ossicles, the *malleus* (or *hammer*), is attached to the eardrum, and when it is set into vibration by a sound wave, it causes the malleus to vibrate. This is connected to the other two ossicles: the *incus* (or *anvil*) and the *stapes* (or *stirrup*), so vibrations are transmitted through them, and passed to the inner ear, via the *oval window,* which is attached to the stapes. The middle ear is connected to the oral cavity by the *eustachian tube,* whose purpose is to ensure an equalization of pressure between the middle and the outer ear. Large pressure differences may distort the eardrum, but if a pressure difference is experienced (e.g. during the ascent or descent of an aeroplane), it can be equalized by swallowing. This has the effect of opening the normally closed eustachian tube, which then equalizes the pressure.

The inner ear is located in the skull, and contains the cochlea. The cochlea has a coiled shell shape, and it is here that physical vibrations are changed to neural impulses, from which the brain can decode the speech signal into its meaningful elements. The cochlea is divided into two sections, called the *scala vestibuli* and the *scala tympani*; it is divided into these sections by two membranes, known as the *vestibular membrane* and the *basilar membrane.* When sound waves arrive at the oval window, they are carried through fluid, called *perilymph,* and cause the basilar membrane to vibrate. The amplitude and the location of vibration of the membrane depends on the frequency of the received sound wave; high frequencies, for example, cause a greater vibration amplitude near the oval window. The final stage of the transformation of sound vibrations into neural impulses occurs in the organ of Corti – an organ consisting of hair cells which sits on the basilar membrane. When the membrane vibrates, the hair cells are set in motion, and nerve fibres from the auditory nerve transmit the vibrations to the auditory centre of the brain. At this point, the brain begins to convert the neural impulses into meaningful phonological units.

Hearing loss

Any damage, disease, or problems occurring in either the peripheral or the internal auditory system may result in some degree of hearing loss, and in some cases, complete deafness. This section briefly describes some different types of hearing impairment.

Hearing loss which is caused by disorders of the outer or middle ear is called *conductive deafness.* Examples of such disorders are the lack of, or damage to the eardrum, or the lack of meatus or pinna. In these cases, the speech signal is prevented, or partially prevented, from being conducted from the outer ear to the inner ear, often because of a congenital disorder. Certain diseases can also cause conductive deafness, e.g. otosclerosis and otitis media. In many cases, however, surgery can rectify the disorder, and where this is not possible, a hearing aid boosts sound levels, making them less faint to the listener.

Hearing loss whose source is damage to the inner ear or auditory nerve is termed *sensorineural deafness* (also *perceptive, neural* or *nerve deafness*). Ménière's disease is an example of a disease causing damage to the auditory nerve, while an inability to hear sounds at high frequencies is an example of hearing loss caused by damage to the receptor cells in the organ of Corti.

A third type of hearing loss is caused by damage to the auditory nerve in the brain stem, or in the cortex, and is known as *central deafness*. This kind of impairment prevents patients from translating the acoustic signal into a meaningful linguistic message.

Audiometry

We have seen that there are different types and different degrees of hearing loss. Audiological measurement, or audiometry, is a technique used to determine the nature and extent of hearing impairment, and this section looks at two audiometric approaches.

Pure tone audiometry

Pure tone audiometry may be used to distinguish between sensorineural and conductive deafness, and also to determine the extent of hearing loss. It involves presenting the subject with pure tones (tones with a single frequency) selected from a spectrum of tones, altering the intensity of the tone, and instructing the subject to indicate the point at which they can just hear the tone. This level at which the tone first becomes audible – the threshold level – is marked on a form called an audiogram and is measured in decibels in relation to what the threshold for that particular tone in a subject with normal hearing would be. The signal is presented separately to each ear, and is fed to the subject either through headphones (air conduction) or by applying the signal to the bone behind the ear (bone conduction).

If the audiogram shows a general lowering of thresholds, across all the frequencies, this suggests that the hearing loss is conductive. If, on the other hand, the threshold levels are lowered to a greater extent in the higher frequencies, this is indicative of sensorineural deafness.

Although pure tone audiometry is a quick and easy method of gauging the type and extent of hearing loss, it does have some disadvantages. The first problem is that pure tones are very different from real speech, since every speech sound has a number of frequencies. The subject's response to real speech can therefore not be predicted with any certainty. Second, the subject is asked to indicate the point at which the sound becomes just audible, and again, this is unhelpful when it comes to assessing how the subject will respond to speech. This is because there is no guarantee that if the sound were a speech sound, they would hear it well enough to make sense of it or to distinguish it from other speech sounds. Finally, the accuracy of the subjects' responses may vary: an overly cautious subject may indicate that he or she hears the sound a few decibels above his threshold level, whereas a less careful one may indicate the actual threshold level. For these reasons, another approach, called *speech audiometry* is sometimes used in addition to, or as an alternative to, pure tone audiometry.

Speech audiometry

In this approach, real speech is used as the stimulus to be presented to the subject, and is presented in such a way that a balance of sounds from the language is used. The subject is then asked to repeat what they have heard, or to select the correct response from a set of similar answers. The audiogram in each case shows the percentage of correctly recognized phrases, words or phonemes at different decibel levels. This method is unsuitable for children, as many of them will be unable to respond to the required tasks.

   Audiometry, then, is a useful tool for audiological measurement, although it has some limitations. It can indicate the type and extent of hearing loss, and in so doing, can predict the likely extent of the subject's language development.

Auditory feedback

If speakers cannot hear themselves speak, they will not be able to monitor their speech as well as speakers with normal hearing. This may be illustrated by the well-known scenario of a person inadvertently shouting while listening to loud music through earphones. The person cannot hear him- or herself speak, and is thus incapable of monitoring the level of loudness of the speech. The ability to hear and monitor one's speech is known as *feedback,* and it is an important factor in auditory phonetics, as feedback is essential for an accurate phonetic output. There are, however, other types of feedback than auditory; two of these will also be described in this section.

   In the case of a normal speaker, speech sounds are fed back to the ear with a delay of approximately 0.001 s. The process of auditory feedback involves the information contained in the speech sound returning to a stage of higher neural planning, where the message is devised and organized into phonological elements, and where the nerve impulses are planned and ordered to produce the speech sound. (See Figure 8.1 for the different stages of activity involved in speech production.) As we can see from the diagram, feedback from the acoustic output to the higher neural planning stage is relatively long. Stop consonants, for example, are likely to be finished by the time they are perceived, meaning that monitoring is impossible. As the example described in the introduction shows, however, auditory feedback is important for monitoring loudness, and also for other suprasegmental features, such as pitch and stress.

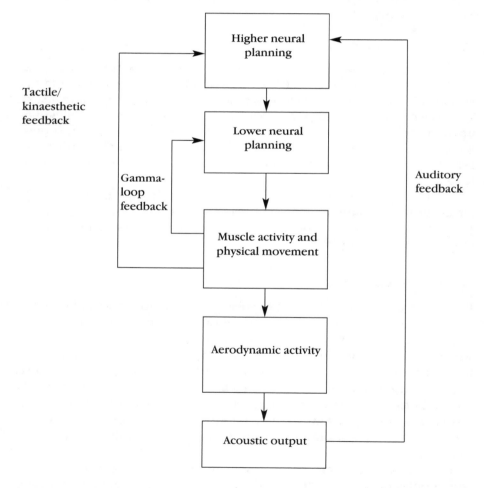

Figure 8.1. Feedback systems. Adapted from Ball (1993).

Tactile and kinaesthetic feedback

Throughout the vocal tract, a series of tactile and kinaesthetic receptors are located. The former provide the speaker with information about touch and pressure, while the latter provide information about the movement, pressure and placement of the various articulators. These are important for the accuracy of both manner and place of articulation, and evidence shows that speakers with an impairment in those receptors may have articulation disorders. The speech production diagram in Figure 8.1 shows that this type of feedback is quicker than auditory feedback, and is thus capable of monitoring a greater number of speech sounds.

Gamma-loop feedback

This type of feedback is capable of monitoring the finer articulatory movements, as it is even quicker than tactile and kinaesthetic feedback (see diagram). This type of feedback involves the neural impulses that originate at higher levels of planning being carried by alpha and gamma motor neurons to the muscles. This results in movement of the muscles, which is sensed in the *muscle spindle.* This sends impulses via the gamma system back to the alpha motor neurons. Then an automatic process causes the returning gamma signal to be compared with the intended outgoing signal, meaning that changes can be made where necessary.

Psychoacoustic experiments

We briefly described above how speech sounds are heard and perceived by the listener. In this section, the way in which types and features of sounds are perceived by the listener and how they are measured are described in more detail. This field of experimentation concerning what listeners can hear is described as *psychoacoustics.* It must, however, be remembered that this is not an exact science, since the listener's response is made on a purely subjective basis.

Psychoacoustic measurements

This section examines the psychoacoustic measurements that are used to measure the perceptions of the various aspects of speech. The first of these aspects is pitch. Pitch is derived from the fundamental frequency, which in turn depends on the frequency of vibration of the vocal folds. Frequency is measured in Hertz, whereas perceived measurements of pitch are made in mels. The *mel* scale is logarithmic, rather than linear, meaning that it does not increase by regular amounts, but by multiplication of units. Hertz measurements are compared with their mel equivalents in Table 8.1. As the scale shows, listeners are more sensitive to pitch changes in the lower frequencies than in the higher ones. The *bark* scale works in a similar way to the mel scale, and is used increasingly in auditory phonetics.

Table 8.1. Pitch and frequency

Pitch (mels)	Frequency (Hz)
0	20
250	160
500	394
750	670
1000	1000
1250	1420
1500	1900
1750	2450
2000	3120
2250	4000

From Ball (1993).

Perceived loudness is measured using the *phon* scale. Unlike the decibel scale, which depends on intensity, this scale allows for the fact that sounds with the same physical intensity, but different frequencies, may be perceived as having different levels of loudness. The *sone* scale is also used to quantify perceived levels of loudness, and works on the basis of a numerical index. For instance, a sound that measures 2 sones is perceived as being twice as loud as one that measures 1 sone.

Experimental procedures

Since the subjective view of what the listener hears is important in this field of phonetics, some thought must go into the type of listener chosen for any particular experiment. It is normally the case that a *naive listener*, i.e. one who has had no phonetics training, is employed. Other aspects that may be important are whether the subject is a foreign or a native speaker, whether the subject is bilingual or monolingual, the age and gender, and possibly even the handedness of the subject.

In carrying out the experiments, four basic types of questions may be asked: *detection, discrimination, identification* and *scaling*. Detection experiments normally concern studies on loudness. In such investigations, the subject is asked to indicate at which point the stimulus can be detected. Discrimination studies involve the subject noticing differences between stimuli. Differences may be in terms of pitch or loudness, or may involve differences between segments. Identification experiments instruct the listener to label certain sounds according to a given set of labels. Scaling tasks ask the subject to place the stimulus along a certain scale, e.g. the mel scale for pitch, or the sone scale for loudness.

The next consideration is the type of stimulus to be presented. In some cases – depending on the type of experiment – natural speech is suitable. In other cases, synthetic speech may be preferable, particularly when precise acoustic cues, which should not be subject to the slight variations that occur in natural speech, are being analysed. The use of synthetic speech means also that slight alterations can be made by the investigator to find out which aspects are important in perception. The investigator may, for example, alter VOT lengths or formant frequencies. From these psychoacoustic experiments, researchers have been able to identify the principal acoustic cues occurring in speech, and these are described in Chapter 6.

Techniques in auditory phonetics

This section examines two techniques and the necessary instrumentation involved in auditory phonetics.

Delayed auditory feedback

As stated in the previous section, auditory feedback in a normal speaker takes approximately 0.001 s (1 ms). Delayed auditory feedback (DAF) is a process which delays the time it takes for the speech signal to be fed back to the ear and thus be perceived by the speaker. The process has both theoretical and practical implications: theoretical in that it provides information as to the role of auditory feedback in speech production, and practical, in that it may be used to remedy disordered speech.

The effects of DAF on normal and disordered speech

DAF has both direct and indirect effects on normal speakers in terms of disruption of their speech. The direct effects include syllable repetitions, mispronunciations, omissions, substitutions and additions. Indirect effects include a slowing of speech tempo, an increase in loudness and an increase in fundamental frequency. Evidence shows that the degree of disruption to speech varies according to the age of the speaker. Mackay (1968) carried out studies on different age groups using several delay times, and it was found that the delay necessary to produce disruption in speech decreases as the age of the speaker increases. For example, children between 4 and 6 years were found to display most disruption when the delay time was 500 ms, while those in the 7–9 age group experienced most disruption at 400 ms. In adults, the peak disruption delay time is 200 ms.

DAF is also used in studies of disordered speech, particularly in cases of stuttering. Studies also exist on speakers with aphasia, apraxia, dysarthria and Parkinson's disease. The reason for concentrating studies on speakers who stutter is that DAF has been proved to reduce or eliminate the disfluency. The length of delay is important, but there seem to be more individual differences than there are in normal speakers. Evidence shows that a stutterer is likely to have a delay time which produces maximum fluency and a longer delay time which produces maximum disruption.

DAF is thus used clinically to treat stuttering, and has had widespread success. A study by Ryan and Van Kirk (1974) describes a step-by-step treatment programme for achieving fluent speech. In the clinic, the speaker is trained to speak for a prolonged period of time in different speaking styles, e.g. reading, conversation, using DAF as an aid. The delay time is initially set at 250 ms, and is gradually reduced by 50 ms at a time, until eventually there is no delay, and the speaker is able to maintain fluent speech, even outside the clinical setting.

Instrumentation

Delays in auditory feedback can be achieved by using a standard reel-to-reel tape recorder with separate playback and record heads. The record head records the speech on to the tape, which then passes to the playback head and is played back to the speaker via headphones. The length of the delay depends on the distance between the heads and the speed of the tape, and this type of device provides four delay times: 80, 160, 330 and 660 ms. Various commercial devices have also been produced in recent years. Examples of these are the Phonic Mirror, which has five playback heads and gives five delay times: 50, 100, 150, 200 and 250 ms. The Aberdeen Speech Aid is another product, and has a continuous range of delay times ranging from 30 to 300 ms. Similar to this is the Danish Phonic Mirror, which has continuous delays from 25 to 220 ms.

Computers may also be used to delay auditory feedback. An example of such a system is PhonX (Phonetic Experimentation) which contains an option to use speech delays from 0 to 1000 ms.

Dichotic listening

Dichotic listening is a technique used in auditory phonetics, and has developed from research carried out in the 1950s (e.g. Broadbent 1954), focusing on the different hearing abilities of the two ears. This section examines the technique of dichotic listening, the instrumentation necessary to achieve it, and its use in studies involving both normal and disordered speech.

Dichotic listening in normal speakers

The technique involves the simultaneous presentation of different auditory material to each ear; material may be verbal (i.e. containing actual speech) or non-verbal (e.g. music, tones). Past studies (e.g. Kimura 1961b, 1964) have shown that normal, right-handed speakers display a right-ear advantage for verbal material and a left-ear advantage for non-verbal material. By *right-ear advantage,* or *left-ear advantage,* it is meant that in dichotic listening tests, the right or left ear forms are heard more often than the opposite ear forms. The auditory pathway which leads from the ear to the opposite hemisphere of the brain is called the *contralateral pathway;* the *ipsilateral pathway* leads to the hemisphere on the same side as the ear. The contralateral pathway is the more efficient of the two, and stops the signal from the ipsilateral pathway. This is why we say that the left hemisphere is more efficient at verbal processing, and that the right is superior when it comes to non-verbal processing. From the findings, it has been inferred that there are differences in the behaviour of the left and right hemispheres of the brain, and researchers have used the technique to find out to what degree hemispheric differences relate to factors such as handedness, gender and age. Bryden and Allard (1978) conclude that hemispheric specialization does not exist at birth, but develops later, and indeed continues to develop throughout life.

Dichotic listening and disordered speech

Dichotic listening studies have been carried out on subjects with disordered speech, particularly aphasic speakers and stutterers. The purpose of such research is to discover whether or not the pattern of left-hemisphere specialization for language has been disturbed – a hypothesis first put forward by Orton (1928) and Travis (1931). Two later studies, however, (Brady and Berson 1975, Dorman and Porter 1975) concluded that only a small percentage of stutterers have a hemispheric organization different from that of normal speakers. Results of these and other studies carried out since are clearly inconsistent, showing that more research is needed in this area.

Studies carried out on aphasic subjects have suggested that the degree of left-ear preference increases with time from the onset of the disorder (see, for example, Pettit and Noll 1979, Crosson and Warren 1981). Past research has also shown that the more severely aphasic the subject, the greater the left-ear preference (e.g. Johnson, Sommers and Weidner

1977). These conclusions suggest that verbal processing shifts from the left to the right hemisphere of the brain, and that this effect increases both with time from the onset of the disorder, and with its severity.

Instrumentation

The instrumentation necessary to prepare a dichotic tape and to carry out a dichotic listening test include: a stereo tape recorder and earphones (to present the material) and two mono reel-to-reel tape recorders, a dual beam storage oscilloscope, microphone and a sound-level meter (to prepare the tape). The signal on the mono tape recorders is adjusted to the required level of equal intensity between the two sounds, and by moving the tape loops, the onset of the two signals are made simultaneous. This is shown by tracings on the oscilloscope. A pair of tokens can then be recorded on to the two channels of the stereo tape recorder, each of which is linked to each ear of the stereo headphones, and is presented to the subject.

Various methods may be used to elicit a response from the subject. First, the type of stimulus to be presented must be established: it may be in the form of words, syllables, tones or environmental sounds. The mode of presentation must then be decided: stimuli can be presented in single pairs and the subject asked for a response, or else several pairs can be presented in quick succession, followed by a pause for the response. Finally, the mode of response is decided. A *forced choice* response may be required, where the subject must choose between one of several pairs presented. Alternatively, *free recall* may be employed, in which case the subject responds with as many of the stimulus items as he or she can remember.

Further reading

Johnson (1997) deals with auditory phonetics and Ryalls (1996) covers speech perception. Code (1997) looks in detail at psychoacoustic experimentation.

CHAPTER 9

Auditory and Perceptual Analysis of Disordered Speech

As described in the previous chapter, the two main forms of auditory phonetic experimentation that have been used in clinical phonetics have been delayed auditory feedback (DAF) and dichotic listening (DL). We feel that the easiest way to illustrate the use of these techniques is to describe some of the classic studies that have employed them: both as an assessment aid, and as a remediation tool.

Delayed auditory feedback

One of the early classic accounts of DAF appeared in Fairbanks and Guttman (1958), and described the effects of DAF on normal speakers. In previous work, Fairbanks (1955) had reported that the effects of DAF on normal speakers had included disturbed articulation and increased durations (what Fairbanks and Guttman term *direct effects* of DAF), and greater sound pressure and higher fundamental frequency (*indirect effects* derived from attempts by the speaker to overcome the DAF). The Fairbanks and Guttman article is an attempt by the authors to detail the articulation disturbance in phonetic terms. They analyse the DAF effects by word for their subjects, and divide the effects into several categories: substitution, omission, addition, and miscellaneous. The measurements are undertaken on a 55-word stretch in the middle of the experimental reading passage. The subjects were 16 young males, who were recorded before DAF was administered, then with headphones with the auditory feedback set at the following delay rates: 0, 0.1, 0.2, 0.4 and 0.8 s (100, 200, 400 and 800 ms), and then again at 0 s.

Looking at the overall measure of correct words, together with correct duration and correct word rate, demonstrated that the 200 ms delay rate corresponded to peak disturbance on these measures. Delays beyond this point showed a decrease in disturbance on the three measures, though they were still more disturbed than zero delay. There were little differences in the scores for the three measures between the initial and post-experimental 0 s recordings, or the pre-experimental recording without headphones.

Turning to the error types, Fairbanks and Guttman note that when the delay was set to the most disruptive level (200 ms) the major error type was addition, followed by substitutions and then omissions. This pattern was similar with the 400 ms delay level, but at 100 ms and 800 ms additions are less common and substitutions and omissions are more or less equally common. The pre-experimental recording and the two 0 s recordings showed very little addition, and a small amount of substitution and omission (omissions were more common than substitutions in the post-experimental recording).

A detailed analysis of the substitutions demonstrated that outside the 200 ms and 400 ms delays, the most common errors were of voicing, affecting only one phoneme in a string, and mostly restricted to unstressed syllables. At the 200 ms and 400 ms level, however, other errors (e.g. place, manner) are almost twice as common as voicing errors, more than one phoneme in a string could be affected (though this is still rare), and stressed syllables are affected more than unstressed.

With omissions, there were no major differences between the delay settings apart from the expected increase in occurrence with the 200 ms and 400 ms settings. Single phoneme omissions predominated in all delay settings, and unstressed syllables were consistently more often affected than stressed.

Additions were divided into repetitions (70% of additions) and insertions. Most of the repetitions involved two articulations covering one or two phonemes. Again, we see that stressed syllables are affected notably more often than unstressed with the two delay settings of 200 ms and 400 ms, although other settings showed a small preference for the stressed syllables as well. With insertions, unstressed syllables are consistently more often affected, with insertions typically consisting of a single phoneme, and occurring more often between than within words.

Fairbanks and Guttman conclude that their study has demonstrated that maximal disturbance in DAF occurs at 200 ms with normal speakers; severity of articulatory disturbance varied between delay settings and between types of error, and the interaction between these two features was also evident. Also, that there was a high incidence of repetitions found at the 200 ms delay level, what has sometimes been termed *artificial stuttering*.

Naturally, the production of artificial stuttering in normal speakers prompted research into DAF with disfluent speakers. Code (1997) reviews much of this work and, as he notes, much interest was generated by

findings that stutterers can often produce fluent speech under DAF conditions. Improvements under DAF usually appear under relatively short time
delays: Sark *et al* (1993) found that improvements in both normal and
rapid reading increased markedly between 25 and 50 ms, with a smaller
decrease in disfluencies up to 75 ms. Code notes that longer delays will
produce disfluencies again, as with normal speakers.

Work has also been undertaken to compare artificial and genuine
stuttering. Although some research suggests the two phenomena are
similar, Code (1997) notes that there is strong evidence to support the
view that they are not identical. Subjective judges are able to distinguish
between genuine and artificial stuttering, and Code himself, in a 1979
study using EMG, showed that there were significant differences in the
muscle activity of the genuine and the artificial stutterer. These differences
suggest that an explanation of the DAF effect on disfluent speakers as
simply one of distraction (in the same way as auditory masking) is
probably too simplistic a view. As Code notes, if DAF is simply a distractor,
then any delay should produce fluency, and this is not what we find.

Many researchers have investigated DAF with disfluent speakers, but
some early and more recent work has also been directed to various
aphasic syndromes. Boller and Marcie (1978) investigated whether
abnormal auditory feedback might play a role in conduction aphasia. At
this time some researchers had begun to investigate the relation between
DAF and different types of aphasia, and it was this initial work that
spurred the authors on in their study. They were especially interested in
conduction aphasia, and hypothesized that conduction aphasics would
show little DAF effect, this being consistent with a view that abnormal
auditory feedback causes some of the features recorded with this type of
aphasia.

The subject, a 63-year-old man, was asked to repeat four monosyllables, one polysyllabic word, and a simple sentence under simultaneous
auditory feedback (SAF) and DAF with a delay of 200 ms. His performance
was compared to 20 controls recorded under identical conditions. Three
different measurements were undertaken.

- First, subjective judgements were obtained from two judges who rated
  the recordings according to changes in intensity, duration, rhythm and
  quality of speech. Overall scores were obtained by adding these
  components together.
- Second, a duration score was obtained by measuring the length of time
  the utterances took under the two conditions (SAF and DAF).
- Finally, a phonemic analysis was undertaken to allow the number of
  phonemic errors to be counted.

In all three of these measures, the controls demonstrated negative effects from DAF. That is to say, their subjective scores showed a marked decrease in overall quality, the duration scores showed increases for monosyllables, the polysyllable and the sentence, and the phonemic analysis showed a mean increase in errors of 8.27. The aphasic patient, on the other hand, showed a remarkably different pattern of results. There was a significantly lower score on the subjective measures, and in fact the subject was judged better under DAF for the polysyllabic word and the sentence. The duration of all the items was decreased under DAF for the subject as opposed to the controls, and the phonemic analysis showed overall fewer errors (−2.6) under DAF than under SAF.

In their discussion of these results, the authors note that speech production relies on two types of feedback: internal phonemic (i.e. the correct selection of phonological features for the sounds about to be uttered), and external phonemic, including auditory feedback. The kinds of production errors found in conduction aphasia suggest that there is impaired encoding (and internal feedback) leading to phonemic paraphrasias. Boller and Marcie also suggest that the results of their study would support a claim that the external auditory feedback is impaired as well with this syndrome. It would appear that auditory feedback is delayed as, under SAF, the subject behaved like normals under DAF. Under DAF, however, the subject improved, echoing the findings of normals when delayed auditory feedback is extended beyond the 200 ms threshold. They conclude, therefore, by suggesting that in conduction aphasia abnormal auditory feedback plays a significant role.

In the final study of this section, Dagenais, Southwood and Mallonnee (1999) looked at DAF in patients with Parkinsonism. The main aims of their study were twofold: first, to investigate in depth the effect of DAF on Parkinsonian speakers as a follow-up to several previous studies; and second, to describe in detail the speech rate reduction noted by previous researchers. The first aim was prompted by differences in findings using DAF with Parkinsonian speakers. With some mildly impaired speakers DAF produced a slowing down of responses; more severely impaired subjects reported elsewhere did not respond to DAF at all. The authors speculate that these differences may be due to differing amounts of limitation on cognitive processing abilities, perhaps coupled to resource allocation problems. In this study the authors investigated three groups of subjects: Parkinsonian speakers of varying degrees of severity, age-matched geriatric controls with no speech problems, and gender-matched normal young adults. Various tasks were undertaken, including reading passages, picture descriptions and spontaneous speech. Three DAF levels were used: 0 ms delay, 125 ms delay and 231 ms delay. Speech samples for all subjects were then scored in terms of speech rate (syllables per minute), articulation rate (fluent syllables per second), fluency (percent fluent syllables) and intelligibility (percentage of correct syllables).

Quite detailed results were produced by Dagenais *et al*, as they were investigating four measures, with three subject groups, in three DAF modes, and of three different speech sample types. Nevertheless, we can summarize their findings as follows. All subject groups showed decreases in the four measures (speech rate, articulation rate, fluency and intelligibility) from 0 DAF to 125 ms and 231 ms. Generally, these decreases were significant when the 0 rate was compared to the two positive DAF rates, but not between 125 ms and 231 ms. Comparing the three groups of subjects, no significant differences were noted on any measure when the DAF was at 0; overall, however, the young adults scored highest and the Parkinsonian group lowest. The differences between the Parkinsonian group and the other two groups were significant for the reading passage in speech rate and articulation rate under the DAF settings. Also, spontaneous speech of the Parkisonian speakers was scored significantly less intelligible than the other groups, but as all scores were high, this could have been due to a ceiling effect. There were no statistically significant differences between the groups for the fluency measure.

The DAF conditions had a negligible effect on intelligibility (as the authors predicted), but did result in significantly reduced rates as speakers attempted to overcome the DAF effect. Some, non-significant, increase in disfluency was evidenced by the Parkinsonian speakers (not expected), and the authors speculate that this may be because the rate reduction was not enough to overcome the DAF. The reading task produced both speech rate and articulation rate reductions in the Parkinsonian group, whereas for the picture description and spontaneous speech only articulation rate reduced noticeably.

Dagenais, Southwood and Mallonnee speculate that the rate reductions may be due to Parkinsonian speakers' difficulties undertaking both a speech production and speech monitoring task simultaneously, or possibly a problem with speech initiation. However, other researchers have shown that Parkinsonian subjects do have problems with resource allocation if required to undertake two tasks. This would also relate to previous findings with severe Parkinsonian subjects referred to above, where they had no resources at all to allocate to speech monitoring and did not respond to DAF. The authors' findings, then, suggest that DAF produces only rate reductions, and not articulatory improvements due to the resource allocation problems already referred to. It is not, therefore, a suitable therapy tool to aid articulation in Parkinsonian speakers.

Dichotic listening

As we saw in the previous chapter, dichotic listening is a technique that has been used to investigate hemispheric dominance in speech perception, for example, through the presentation of series of digits binaurally, with a different digit presented simultaneously to each ear. Naturally, such a technique lends itself well to the investigation of aphasia. An early study reporting dichotic listening effects with aphasic speakers is reported in Sparks, Goodglas and Nickel (1970), although the earliest work in the area dates back to Broadbent (1954) and Kimura (1961a, b). As Sparks, Goodglas and Nickel note, previous work had reported a cerebral dominance effect of 2–6% in correctness of report from digits presented to the right ear for normal right-handed subjects in dichotic tests. This dominance pattern was altered in speakers with temporal lobe lesions, adding a deficit of about 8% to the ear contralateral to the lesion. Work with other patient types and with temporal lobe removal showed further patterns of deficit; indeed, temporal lobe removal produced more severe impairments to both ears if the left temporal lobe was removed than if it was the right.

Sparks, Goodglas and Nickel (1970) attempt to explain some of the results that were found, bearing in mind the variety of pathways used to take input from the ear to the brain. As shown in Figure 9.1 there are both contralateral (i.e. crossing) pathways from left ear to right hemisphere and right ear to left hemisphere and ipsilateral pathways from left ear to left hemisphere and right ear to right hemisphere. Further, there is a transcallosal pathway for linguistic input from the right hemisphere across the corpus callosum to the left hemisphere.

Previous work on dichotic listening in normals suggested a model (as proposed by Sparks and Geschwind (1968) in which, under dichotic listening conditions, the ipsilateral input is virtually suppressed by the contralateral, and that there is competition in the left hemisphere between input from the right ear arriving via the contralateral pathway, and from the left ear arriving via the transcallosal pathway from the right hemisphere. As the transcallosal pathway involves one extra synaptic step, it is normally the case that the contralateral pathway dominates; indeed, in patients who have had callosal section only right ear input is available for report as the transcallosal pathway is no longer in existence.

Sparks, Goodglas and Nickel (1970) report data from nearly 50 right-handed subjects in an attempt to test and refine the model referred to earlier. The subjects were all male: 28 left brain damaged and 20 right brain damaged. The dichotic listening task involved the subjects repeating what they heard of two sets of input: 20 pairs of digits and 20 pairs of animal names (monosyllables). The results showed the expected pattern,

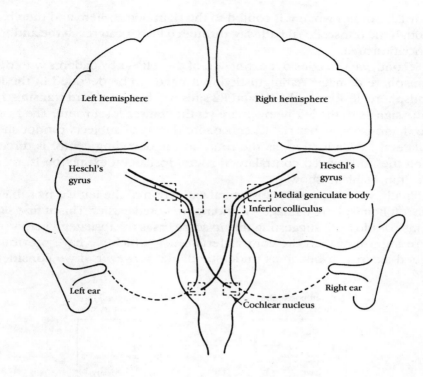

Figure 9.1. Ipsilateral and contralateral pathways from the ears to the brain (Adapted from Code 1997).

whereby the ear contralateral to the cortical injury loses effectiveness. However, the two hemisphere groups did not show exactly the same patterns: the difference between the ears is greater for the right hemisphere impaired subjects than for the left hemisphere group. This was accounted for by the fact that many of the left hemisphere group also demonstrated inferior performance in the ear ipsilateral to their lesion.

The authors explain their findings in terms of their refined model, which is illustrated in Figure 9.2. This figure is an expansion of Figure 9.1 through the addition of a series of possible left and right lesion sites (L1–L3, R1–R2). We can now look at the three different 'extinction' patterns found. First, extinction of the right ear by patients with left hemisphere damage can be accounted for by lesions in the L1 or L2 locations. The diagram shows that the contralateral pathways are dominant, therefore, lesions L1 and L2 stop the signal from arriving in the primary auditory area or the adjacent auditory association area. Input from the left ear is affected through the ipsilateral pathway with lesions at

L1 or L2, but not when it is routed to the right hemisphere and then back through the transcallosal pathway, through which it can reach the auditory association area.

Second, we can consider extinction of the left ear by patients with right hemisphere damage. As linguistic input needs to be decoded in the left hemisphere, lesions in the R1 and R2 sites will block onward transmission of the signals to the left hemisphere via the transcallosal route. The figure also demonstrates that right hemisphere damaged subjects cannot show ipsilateral ear extinction, as the route to the decoding centre is directly along the undamaged contralateral route. Ipsilateral extinction is, therefore, impossible to show.

Finally, we can consider ipsilateral extinction of the left ear by subjects with left hemisphere damage – a finding we noted earlier. This at first sight seems paradoxical, suggesting that in some cases the ipsilateral pathway is more important than the contralateral one – which we have previously argued against. It becomes understandable, however, if we consider a

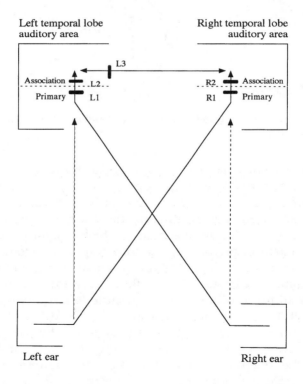

Figure 9.2. Lesions affecting different pathways (Adapted from Code 1997).

lesion at site L3. This would leave input from the right ear via the contra-lateral pathway unaffected, but would disrupt left ear input, as it could not be passed back from the right hemisphere via the corpus callosum.

In their account Sparks, Goodglas and Nickel (1970) have posited a refined model of left and right hemisphere processing of left and right ear input, based on dichotic listening with different brain damaged subjects. In a study of 1979, Damasio and Damasio returned to this topic in an attempt to locate those lesions that cause different ear extinction types as described by Sparks *et al.* They investigated 20 subjects, some with left and some with right hemisphere lesions. They undertook a dichotic listening test and divided the subjects into those showing left ear extinc-tion, those with right ear extinction and those with normal dichotic listening results. Of the eight who showed left ear extinction, four had left hemisphere and four right hemisphere lesions. Of course, of primary interest in terms of the Sparks *et al* model were those subjects with left ear extinction and left hemisphere damage. All subjects were investigated through the use of computerized axial tomography, which allowed the sites of lesions to be studied in detail. The subjects with left ear extinction and left hemisphere lesions were looked at in order to ascertain a likely pathway for the interhemispheric link. Their findings suggest that such a connection must lie outside the geniculocortical pathways, and that the auditory fibres are outside the optical radiations but in close relationship with them (Damasio and Damasio 1979, p. 653).

We can now turn to an example of the use of dichotic listening as a therapy tool. The experiment reported in Code (1989) was prompted by a large body of work on hemispheric specialization. As Code notes, there is a general agreement that the two hemispheres of the brain are specialized for different tasks – the left is often characterized as superior for linguistic-analytic cognitive processing, with the right better in holistic-Gestalt processing. However, the extent of this specialization has been a matter of debate, as has the amount to which certain processing tasks could shift hemispheres as a result, for example, of hemispheric damage.

Code refers to evidence both from studies of normal subjects (e.g. through studying cerebral blood flow, or dichotic listening tasks), and from aphasic subjects (e.g. hemispherectomy patients who recover some language), that 'lateral shift' can occur. If the right hemisphere can take over some of the linguistic functions of the left, is it possible to encourage this to happen more quickly through hemispheric retraining programmes? In this study Code explores three experimental programmes to test this proposal.

It was decided to investigate the effects of hemispheric specialization retraining (HSR) on comprehension in this study, so the subject chosen was a Wernicke's patient. The subject was a 37-year-old male, who had received 3.5 years of speech therapy after a thromboembolic cerebrovascular attack four years previously. A computer tomography (CT) scan confirmed a left temporal lobe lesion. He was judged to have maximized recovery, so could act as his own control for the experimental procedures.

A variety of language tests (including the PICA, BDAE, Revised Token Test, Reporter's Test, and the Digit Span Test) were administered prior to the HSR, and again following the three parts of the HSR. Tests were also carried out to ascertain lateral preference for linguistic material and to rule out right hemisphere damage.

Code notes that important factors in auditory comprehension are phonemic discrimination, auditory verbal retention, and semantic discrimination. Therefore, an HSR promoting right-hemisphere abilities in these areas should result in improvements in the subject's communicative abilities.

The HSR consisted of three parts (each lasting just over six months). Part 1 involved dichotic listening. The tapes prepared for this part had a phonemic discrimination section (to discriminate voicing, place and voicing plus place in stop + /ɑ/ syllables); a digit section with pauses to test auditory retention; and a CVC section with pauses to test both discrimination and retention.

Part 2 used the tachistoscopic hemifield viewing method to present visual-verbal material simultaneously to the left and right visual field. The tasks included letter, digit, and CVC identification, and semantic discrimination via an odd-one-out task. Part 3 combined these approaches with material presented both aurally and visually at the same time. For all these parts, the subject had to report what he heard in the left ear, or saw in the left visual field (corresponding to the right hemisphere).

The results of the post-HSR linguistic tests showed a significant improvement in general communicative ability, modest changes in both non-redundant comprehension of language and in verbal fluency, and a great increase in ability in the auditory retention of digits. Laterality tests before the HSR had shown left ear, left visual field dominance (suggesting the right hemisphere had already begun to take over linguistic processing). After training, this pattern was strengthened.

Code points out that the study does not conclusively prove that the subject demonstrated lateral shift for language processing, as the experimental design did not preclude material arriving at the right hemisphere being moved to the left for processing (although, in this case, this would seem unlikely due to the lesion). Nevertheless, this is an interesting study, showing the possibility of using dichotic listening as a therapy tool as well as an assessment technique.

Further reading

A straightforward introduction to speech perception is supplied by Ryalls (1996), and this area is also covered in Ball (1993) and Ball and Rahilly (1999). Code (1997) provides an in-depth examination of instrumental and experimental issues in speech perception.

CHAPTER 10

The Future of Clinical Phonetics

One of the questions that is frequently asked about future developments in phonetics is whether it will soon be possible to have some kind of automatic transcription machine: that is to say, a device into which we could play the speech of the subject under investigation, and from which we could obtain a printed transcription into IPA. For clinical purposes, obviously, this would need to be a narrow transcription for reasons discussed in Chapter 3. Most people envisage this to be an acoustic analysis device, something like a sound spectrograph linked to an IPA database. This database would contain ideal acoustic patterns for individual sounds and could then match these to the incoming signal.

There are, however, major problems with this concept.

- First, the amount of acoustic detail one would need to scan to get a narrow transcription sits uneasily with the amount of flexibility the system needs to get round all those acoustic features that are derived from the speaker's individual vocal tract, and those that are derived from the particular speech event (i.e. loudness, tempo), and which are, therefore, non-linguistic and need to be filtered out.
- Second, there is the problem of boundaries: IPA symbols suggest that segments have clearly defined boundaries but, as we have noted elsewhere, this is not reflected in the acoustic record. It will not, therefore, be easy to have a system that aligns artificial segment boundaries with the varying acoustic boundaries of voice, friction, burst release of stops, etc.
- Third, and perhaps most importantly, we must recall what was described in Chapter 5, that the acoustic record does not always correspond exactly with the articulatory posture. Several EPG studies have shown, for example, that fronting of velar stops to alveolar stops (as it would appear from both impressionistic transcription, and acoustic analysis) may well be more complex. It seems that subjects produce

target alveolars more or less correctly, whereas the target velars have a double articulation consisting of both alveolar and velar contacts overlapping in time. However, because the alveolar contact is released after that velar one, it sounds as if the subject has produced a simple alveolar stop.

Currently, therefore, we see no immediate possibility of a device to convert acoustic signals into IPA transcription at a level of detail that would be of use to the clinical phonetician. If acoustic devices are not immediately feasible, could we produce an articulatory device that could do the job? We have seen how, in order to get a complete picture of speech production, we use a range of instruments: EMG to measure muscle activity, ELG/EGG to investigate vocal fold activity, aerometry and naso-metry to examine airflows in the vocal tract, and EPG to look at tongue–palate contact. Someone wired up to all (or even several) of these at once would be a formidable sight, and would be unlikely to be producing very natural speech! Even using all these instruments, we should probably still need acoustic information (to tell us about vowels, for example).

The one possible advance towards such a goal comes from the devel-opment in imaging techniques reported in Chapter 4. If we could combine a three-dimensional, real-time imaging system with acoustic analysis and link this to some kind of interpretative module that could fit transcriptions to the combination of acoustic and articulatory data, we might then get our automatic transcription machine. Radiographic techniques are too dangerous, MRI machinery is too big and expensive and ultrasound too localized, but recent developments in the design of electromagnetic articulography (EMA) equipment suggest that a more manageable system may eventually be available and so could form part of such an endeavour.

In the meantime, what instances do we have at the moment of combining techniques? We shall look in the next few pages at examples of combining electrolaryngography with laryngoscopy; electropalatography and acoustic analysis, EPG and nasometry, and EMA with acoustic data.

Combining techniques

Electrolaryngography (ELG) is an indirect method of measuring vocal fold activity, as we noted in Chapter 4. On the other hand, laryngoscopy is a direct method of seeing and photographing the larynx using a rigid or flexible endoscope. ELG, however, provides numerical data, allowing us to derive a range of useful measures that can tell us about pitch changes in the voice, and how well a person's voice matches normal expectations. If we can combine these two techniques we can match the vocal fold activity to the scores, and can see with laryngoscopy what the folds actually look like, and so spot any irregularities that might be contributing to the ELG findings. Abberton and Fourcin (1997) describe just such a combined approach, using a stroboscopic light connected to the endoscope to aid production of clear views of the vocal folds. Figure 10.1 shows normal and pathological voice (bilateral sulci) production, with the stroboscopic images above the Lx waveforms of the laryngograph. The unusual shape of the Lx waveforms for the pathological speaker are illuminated when we see that the pathological speaker never achieves complete glottal closure.

EPG has been combined with acoustic data on many occasions (Figure 10.2 shows EPG, acoustic, and airflow data). We can briefly look at just three studies, one of which is overtly therapy-oriented. Hoole *et al* (1989) examined the fricative consonants /s/ and /ʃ/ with EPG, at the same time taking acoustic measurements. They wanted to discover the links between acoustic characteristics of fricatives and the tongue gestures that coincide with them. In this way, they hoped to work towards a clinically useful diagnostic routine. An ultimate goal of their research was to see whether one could predict the acoustic characteristics of a sound by looking at the EPG contact patterns during its production. The fricatives were produced by two different speakers, were in two different word positions (initial and medial), and in two different vowel contexts (/i/ and /a/). Examining the different tokens, the authors found that EPG and acoustic analysis were comparable in their sensitivity to these differences. They also found that certain acoustic parameters could indeed be predicted from EPG patterns.

Howard and Varley (1996) used EPG and acoustic measures to investigate a case of severe acquired apraxia of speech. Their initial impressionistic transcriptions had suggested the subject used a range of atypical (for English) articulations, e.g. /n/ being realized as [n], [nj], [ɲ], or [ŋ]. The EPG patterns clarified this by showing that the speaker's gestures were basically alveolar, but variably spread right across the palate to the palatal or velar regions. The acoustic data clarified some of the problems found in transcribing voicing and duration, and when the two techniques were compared, it became clear that closure for intervocalic stops did not (as with normals) last throughout the period of intervocalic silence. The closure was in place for only the latter stages of this intervocalic silence.

Dew, Glaister and Roach (1989) describe an overtly therapeutic combination of EPG and acoustic information. They wished to construct a feedback device that could inform patients of both place and manner of articulation. They divided manner into broad categories (stop, nasal, fricative, vowel, etc.) that could be automatically recognized by computer. This

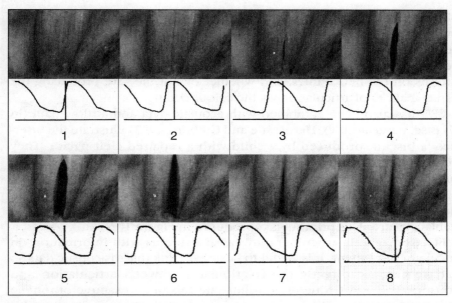

(a) Normal

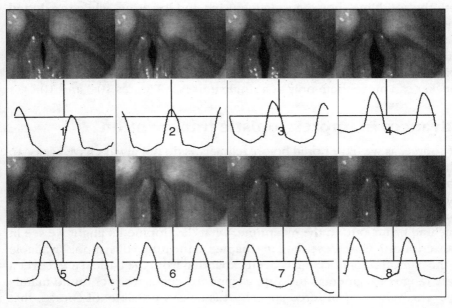

(b) Pathological

Figure 10.1. Electrolaryngography with laryngoscopy (From Abberton and Fourcin 1997).

colour-codes the types (plosive burst, red; nasal, blue; fricative, yellow; vowel, green; and silence, white). These colours are then overlaid on to the EPG frames (this requires a sample rate of about 100 palates per second). The patient can then see both their tongue–palate contact patterns on the EPG frames, and whether or not they are producing the correct manner of articulation via the colour coding.

EPG has also been combined with acoustic data and airflow data (in this case, nasal airflow). Hardcastle and Gibbon (1997) illustrate the utterance 'a biscuit' produced by a child with a repaired cleft palate. They produce a set of EPG frames, together with an acoustic waveform and linked nasal airflow trace. The combined data allow us to note that there was an amount of non-normal nasal airflow during the oral consonants /b/ and /s/ and, further, that the /b/ was accompanied by velar as well as bilabial closure. This printout is reproduced in Figure 10.2.

Electromagnetic articulography can provide us with information on articulator movement. It is useful to be able to link this to acoustic data so that we can see directly the relationship between articulation and acoustics. Ball and Gröne (1997) illustrate this in an example of tongue movement patterns with a normal and a dysarthric speaker. The A and B parts of the diagrams illustrate tongue tip and tongue blade respectively, with the solid line showing tongue raising and lowering, while the dotted line shows tongue movement velocity. The C part links these movements to the acoustic waveform, so we can readily identify where in the test utterance the tongue movements take place. The normal speaker shows an ability to move the tip and blade independently, whereas the dysarthric speaker can move them only as a single unit (see Figures 10.3 and 10.4).

Advances in impressionistic transcription

Of course, as we have noted before, clinicians do not always have access to what can be expensive and complex instrumentation. Therefore, impressionistic transcription will long remain an important tool in their armoury, and even if we ever get an automatic transcription device, clinical phoneticians will still need to know the IPA in order to understand what the machine prints out. In the meantime, what developments might we see in transcription? As we described in Chapter 3, the range of symbols available to the clinical phonetician has been expanded from the basic IPA to cover a wide range of segmental and suprasegmental characteristics found mainly or exclusively in disordered speech. It is always possible, of course, that we may need to add one or two more over the years, but it is hard to see the necessity for major changes in the symbol set.

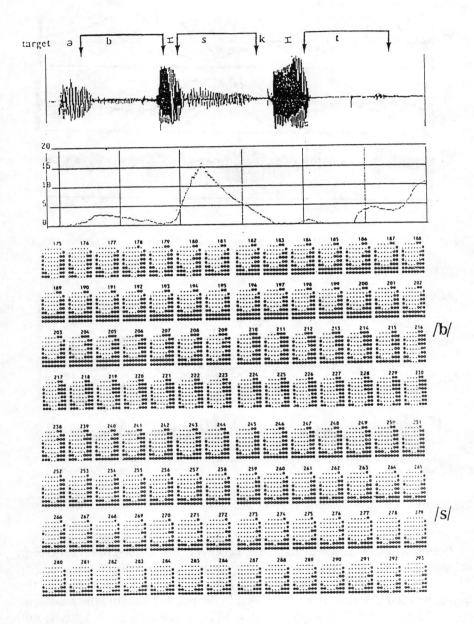

Figure 10.2. EPG with nasal airflow and acoustic waveform (From Hardcastle and Gibbon 1997).

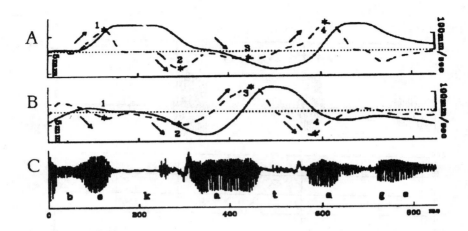

Figure 10.3. EMA with acoustic data – normal speaker (From Ball and Gröne 1997).

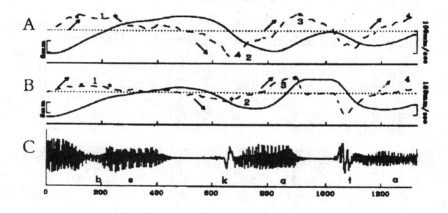

Figure 10.4. EMA with acoustic data – dysarthric speaker (From Ball and Gröne 1997).

Other areas of development are, however, possible. These centre on reliability issues and teaching techniques (which, of course, are linked). There is research (e.g. Shriberg and Lof 1991) which suggests that the more detailed a transcriber is required to be, the less reliable the transcription is likely to be. Reliability was discussed in Chapter 3, and we should remember that it can be measured both between transcribers (inter-transcriber reliability), and for one transcriber across time (intra-transcriber reliability). Both these measures suffer when we ask for increased detail. However, we might also expect that in clinical transcriptions, reliability might improve once we have provided symbols for atypical speech productions which previously had no dedicated IPA symbol.

Clearly this might be the case if we also improve the way we teach the symbol systems. There is no getting round the fact that a lot of time is needed in small classes to introduce the IPA and other related systems to students and to train them in their use. However, we are beginning to see the development of self-learning packages using audio, video and CD-ROM technologies that should be able to cut down this time requirement to some extent. We clearly need a study comparing different teaching techniques on transcribers' reliability scores, and another one comparing their scores when using just the IPA, and when the extIPA and/or VoQS is added in. Such studies will go a long way to guiding our training schedules in the future.

Clinical phonetics, as we see it, is not, however, a simply mechanistic discipline. We are not solely concerned with description of disordered speech behaviours. Any area of study worth pursuing is interested in attempts at explanation as well as description. Clinical phonetics, as well as clinical linguistics, has contributed and will continue to do so, to the debates surrounding models of speech production and perception. Kent (1996), for example, has pointed out how detailed studies of the phonetics of various acquired disorders have informed our understanding of the different components in the speech production mechanism, and which ones, and to which extent, are impaired in disorders such as apraxia of speech, dysarthria and, for example, conduction aphasia. This sort of work has lead us to an understanding that a basic phonetics–phonology model of speech production is too simplistic; we require at least a three-way system with a 'cognitive phonetics' (or organizational) module intervening (see Code and Ball 1988), and these levels interact in disordered speech (see Figure 10.5).

Work reported by Onslow and colleagues (see Packman *et al* 1996) have used detailed studies of the phonetics of disfluency to propose an account of this phenomenon. They describe their approach as the 'Variability Model' (Vmodel) of stuttering. Drawing on previous work, the authors claim that prosody is important in stuttering. In particular, syllabic stress has been the focus of a variety of studies. Packman *et al* have looked at one aspect of syllabic stress: that of vowel duration.

The authors' work suggests that stuttering reduces when the variability of syllabic stress reduces. They interpret their findings in the light of Zimmerman's (1980) suggestion that the speech motor systems of people who stutter are particularly susceptible to variability. It can be argued,

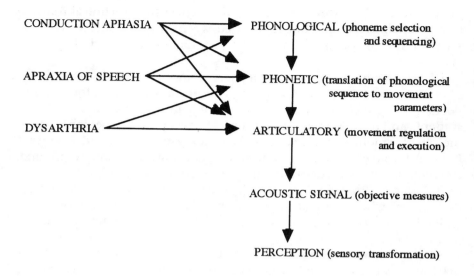

Figure 10.5. Kent model of Speech Organization and Disorders (Adapted from Kent 1996).

then, that the production of syllabic stress contrasts is a source of variability which disrupts the speech systems of these susceptible individuals, and this is why reduction in stress variability is accompanied by reduction in stuttering.

This claim needs to be viewed in the light of what we know about the associations between stress and speech motor control. Stressed syllables demand an increase in neural excitation and muscular exertion that is manifest in an increase in the velocity, extent and duration of displacement of various structures in the vocal tract. In other words, when a syllable is stressed, movements of the structures associated with respiration, phonation and articulation are faster and larger and last longer. Therefore, as Figure 10.6 shows, the production of syllables with a range of stress would require continual and rapid physiological changes, and so is a dynamic, unpredictable, and ever-present source of variability within the speech motor system.

Working from these assumptions, Packman *et al* developed the Vmodel. This suggests that stuttering will decrease when the person reduces stress contrasts. The Vmodel was developed by the authors from the findings of a range of their acoustic research which showed that after certain stuttering treatments, subjects decreased the range of vowel durations during their spontaneous speech. This suggests to the authors

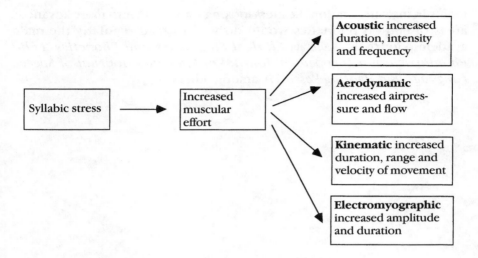

Figure 10.6. Vmodel of stuttering (Adapted from Packman *et al* 1996).

that persons who stutter may be able to decrease their stuttering by decreasing the amount of stress contrast in their speech.

As Figure 10.6 shows, a range of acoustic and physiological instrumentation can be brought to bear in a study of syllabic stress. Acoustic procedures are particularly suited for the measurement of duration (though intensity of the signal could also be examined). Moreover, it is clear that if we wish to examine vowel length in anything more than a cursory manner, instrumental as opposed to impressionistic description has to be used.

Packman *et al* (1996) conclude their sketch of the Vmodel of stuttering by suggesting that stuttering is triggered by the variability inherent in the production of syllabic stress, but in everyday speaking situations the threshold for that triggering is likely to be influenced by emotional and cognitive factors.

Clinical phonetics is, then, not just a tool for the clinician, but also a vital aspect of the search for understanding how speech works. We hope that the readers of this book will find much to help them in the application of phonetics to the clinical situation, but will also contribute to the developments in models of speech production and perception.

Further reading

The sources referred to in this chapter are a good starting place to explore ideas about models of speech production and perception and developments in instrumentation. Readers looking for a route into more advanced areas of clinical phonetics would do well to read regularly the main academic journals, such as *Clinical Linguistics and Phonetics, Folia Phoniatrica and Logopedica, Journal of Phonetics, Journal of Speech Language and Hearing Research,* among others.

References

Abercrombie D (1967) Elements of General Phonetics. Edinburgh: Edinburgh University Press.

Abberton E, Fourcin A (1997) Electrolaryngography. In Ball MJ, Code C (eds), Instrumental Clinical Phonetics, pp. 119–148. London: Whurr.

Ansell BM, Kent RD (1992) Acoustic-phonetic contrasts and intelligibility in the dysarthria associated with mixed cerebral palsy. Journal of Speech Language and Hearing Research, 35: 296–308.

Awan S, Bressman T, Sader R, Horch H (1999) Measures of RMS nasalance using NasalView in patients undergoing secondary osteoplasty. In Maassen B, Groenen P (eds), Pathologies of Speech and Language: Advances in Clinical Phonetics and Linguistics, pp. 333–341. London: Whurr.

Baer T, Gore J, Boyce S, Nye P (1987) Application of MRI to the analysis of speech production. Magnetic Resonance Imaging, 5: 1–7.

Baer T, Gore J, Boyce S, Nye P (1991) Analysis of vocal tract shape and dimensions using magnetic resonance imaging: vowels. Journal of the Acoustical Society of America, 90: 799–828.

Ball MJ (1993) Phonetics for Speech Pathology, 2nd edition. London: Whurr.

Ball MJ, Code C (Eds) (1997) Instrumental Clinical Phonetics. London: Whurr.

Ball MJ, Esling J, Dickson C (1999) Transcription of voice. In Kent RD and Ball MJ (eds) Voice Quality Measurement, pp. 49–58. San Diego: Singular Publishing.

Ball MJ, Gibbon F (eds) (2001) Vowels and Vowel Disorders. Woburn, Mass. Butterworth-Heinemann.

Ball MJ, Gracco V and Stone M (2001) Imaging techniques for the investigation of normal and disordered speech production. Advances in Speech-Language Pathology, 3: 13–25.

Ball MJ, Local J (1996) Advances in impressionistic transcription of disordered speech. In Ball MJ and Duckworth M (eds), Advances in Clinical Phonetics, pp. 51–89. Amsterdam: John Benjamins.

Ball MJ, Gröne B (1997) Imaging techniques. In Ball MJ and Code C (eds), Instrumental Clinical Phonetics, pp. 194–227. London: Whurr.

Ball MJ, Rahilly J (1996) Acoustic analysis as an aid to the transcription of an example of disfluent speech. In Ball MJ and Duckworth M (eds), Advances in Clinical Phonetics, pp. 197–216. Amsterdam: John Benjamins.

Ball MJ, Rahilly J (1999) Phonetics: The Science of Speech. London: Arnold.

Ball MJ, Rahilly J, Tench P (1996) The Phonetic Transcription of Disordered Speech. San Diego: Singular.

Ball MJ, Code C, Rahilly J, Hazlett D (1994) Non-segmental aspects of disordered speech: Developments in transcription. Clinical Linguistics and Phonetics, 8: 67–83.

Boller F, Marcie P (1978) Possible role of abnormal auditory feedback in conduction aphasia. Neuropsychologia, 16: 521–524.

Bowman SA, Shanks JC (1978) Velopharyngeal relationships of /i/ and /s/ as seen cephalometrically for persons with suspected incompetence. Journal of Speech and Hearing Disorders, 43: 185–91.

Bradford A, Dodd B (1996) Do all speech-disordered children have motor deficits? Clinical Linguistics and Phonetics, 10: 77–101.

Brady JP, Berson J (1975) Stuttering, dichotic, listening and cerebral dominance. Archives of General Psychiatry, 32: 1449–52.

Branderud P (1985) Movetrack: a movement tracking system. Proceedings of the French-Swedish Symposium on Speech, 22–24 April 1985, pp. 113–22. Grenoble: GALF.

Broadbent D (1954) The role of auditory localization in attention and memory span. Journal of Experimental Psychology, 47: 191–196.

Bryden MP, Allard F (1978) Dichotic listening and the development of linguistic processes. In Kinsbourne M (ed.) Asymmetrical Function of the Brain. Cambridge: Cambridge University Press.

Carney E (1979) Inappropriate abstraction in speech assessment procedures. British Journal of Disorders of Communication, 14: 123–135.

Catford J (1988) A Practical Introduction to Phonetics. Oxford: Oxford University Press.

Clark J, Yallop C (1995) An Introduction to Phonetics and Phonology, 2nd edition. Oxford: Blackwell.

Code C (1979) Genuine and artificial stammering: an EMG comparison. British Journal of Disorders of Communication, 14: 5–16.

Code C (1989) Hemispheric specialization retraining in aphasia: possibilities and problems. In Code C, Müller D (eds), Aphasia Therapy, 2nd edition. London: Whurr.

Code C (1997) Experimental audioperceptual techniques. In Ball MJ, Code C (eds), Instrumental Clinical Phonetics, pp. 228–261. London: Whurr.

Code C, Ball MJ (1982) Fricative production in Broca's aphasia: a spectrographic analysis. Journal of Phonetics, 10: 325–31.

Code C, Ball MJ (1988) Apraxia of speech: the case for a cognitive phonetics. In Ball MJ (ed) Theoretical Linguistics and Disordered Language, pp. 152–167. London: Croom Helm.

Collins M, Rosenbek JC, Wertz RT (1983) Spectrographic analysis of vowel and word duration in apraxia of speech. Journal of Speech Language and Hearing Research, 26: 224–230.

Coventry K, Clibbens J, Cooper M (1998) The testing and evaluation of a new visual speech aid incorporating digital kymography. In Ziegler W, Deger K (eds), Clinical Phonetics and Linguistics, pp. 501–509. London: Whurr.

Crosson R, Warren RL (1981) Dichotic ear preferences for CVC words in Wernicke's and Broca's aphasia. Cortex, 17: 249–258.

Crystal D, Varley R (1998) Introduction to Language Pathology, 4th edition. London: Whurr.

Dagenais P, Southwood MH, Mallonee K (1999) Assessing processing skills in speakers with Parkinson's disease using delayed auditory feedback. Journal of Medical Speech-Language Pathology, 4: 297–313.

Damasio H, Damasio A (1979) 'Paradoxic' ear extinction in dichotic listening: possible anatomic significance. Neurology, 29: 644–653.

Dang J, Honda K, Suzuki H (1993) MRI measurement and acoustic investigation of the nasal and paranasal cavities. Journal of the Acoustical Society of America, 94: 1765.

Darley F, Aronson A, Brown J (1975) Motor Speech Disorders. Philadelphia: W. B. Saunders.

Demolin D, George M, Lecuit V, Metens T, Soquet A, Raeymakers H (1997) Coarticulation and articulatory compensations studied by dynamic MRI. Proceedings of the 5th European Conference on Speech Communication and Technology, Rhodes, Greece, 43–46.

Denes P, Pinson E (1973) The Speech Chain. New York: Anchor.

Dew A, Glaister N, Roach P (1989) Combining displays of EPG and automatic segmentation of speech for clinical purposes. Clinical Linguistics and Phonetics, 3: 71–80.

Dodd B (ed) (1995) Differential Diagnosis of Children with Speech Disorder. London: Whurr.

Dorman MF, Porter RJ (1975) Hemispheric lateralization for speech perception in stutterers. Cortex, 11: 95–102.

Duckworth M, Allen G, Hardcastle W, Ball MJ (1990) Extensions to the International Phonetic Alphabet for the transcription of atypical speech. Clinical Linguistics and Phonetics, 4: 273–80.

Duffy JR, Gawle CA (1984) Apraxic speakers' vowel duration in consonant–vowel–consonant syllables. In Rosenbak JC, McNeil MR, Aronson AE (eds) Apraxia of Speech: Physiology, Acoustics, Linguistics, Management, pp. 167–196. San Diego: College-Hill Press.

Edwards S, Miller N (1989) Using EPG to investigate speech errors and motor agility in a dyspraxic person. Clinical Linguistics and Phonetics, 3: 111–126.

Enany NM (1981) A cephalometric study of the effects of primary osteoplasty in unilateral cleft lip and palate individuals. Cleft Palate Journal, 18: 286–292.

Fairbanks G (1955) Selective vocal effects of delayed auditory feedback. Journal of Speech and Hearing Disorders, 20: 333–346.

Fairbanks G, Guttman N (1958) Effects of delayed auditory feedback upon articulation. Journal of Speech Language and Hearing Research, 1: 12–22.

Farmer A (1997) Spectrography. In Ball MJ, Code C (eds), Instrumental Clinical Phonetics, pp. 22–63. London: Whurr.

Foldvik A, Kristiansen U, Kværness J, Bonnaventure H (1993) A time-evolving three-dimensional vocal tract model by means of magnetic resonance imaging (MRI). Proceedings Eurospeech 1993, 1: 557–558.

Foldvik A, Kristiansen U, Kvarness J, Torp A, Torp H (1995) Three-dimensional ultrasound and magnetic resonance imaging: a new dimension in phonetic research. Proceedings of the 13th International Congress of Phonetic Sciences, Vol. 4, pp. 46–49. Stockholm: KTH and Stockholm University.

Fry D (1979) The Physics of Speech. Cambridge: Cambridge University Press.

Gibbon F (1990) Lingual activity in two speech-disordered children's attempts to produce velar and alveolar stop consonants: evidence from electropalatographic (EPG) data. British Journal of Disorders of Communication, 25: 329–340.

Gibbon F, Hardcastle W (1989) Deviant articulation in a cleft palate child following late repair of the hard palate: a description and remediation procedure using electropalatography (EPG). Clinical Linguistics and Phonetics, 3: 93–110.

Glaser ER, Skolnick, ML, McWilliams BT, Shprintzen RJ (1979) The dynamics of Passavantís Ridge in subjects with and without velopharyngeal insufficiency: a multi-view video-fluoroscopy study. Cleft Palate Journal, 16: 24–33.

Greenwood A, Goodyear C, Martin P (1992) Measurement of vocal tract shapes using MRI. IEEE Proceedings 1 (Communication, Speech, Vision), 139: 553–560.

Hardcastle W, Gibbon F (1997) Electropalatography and its clinical applications. In Ball MJ, Code C (eds), Instrumental Clinical Phonetics, pp. 149–193. London: Whurr.

Healey EC, Ramig PR (1986) Acoustic measures of stutterers' and non-stutterers' fluency in two speech contexts. Journal of Speech and Hearing Research, 29: 325–31.

Hirose H, Kiritani S, Ushijima T, Sawashima M (1978) Analysis of abnormal articulatory dynamics in two dysarthric patients. Journal of Speech and Hearing Disorders, 43: 96–105.

Hirose H, Kiritani S, Ushijima T, Yoshioka H, Sawshima M (1981) Patterns of dysarthric movements in patients with Parkinsonism. Folia Phoniatrica, 33: 204–15.

Holm A, Dodd B (1999) Differential diagnosis of phonological disorder in two bilingual children acquiring Italian and English. Clinical Linguistics and Phonetics, 13: 113–129.

Hoole P, Ziegler W, Hartmann E, Hardcastle W (1989) Parallel electropalatographic and acoustic measures of fricatives. Clinical Linguistics and Phonetics, 3: 59–69.

Howard S (1993) Articulatory constraints on a phonological system: a case study of cleft palate speech. Clinical Linguistics and Phonetics, 7: 299–317.

Howard S (1998) A perceptual and palatographic case study of Pierre Robin Sequence. In Ziegler W, Deger K (eds), Clinical Phonetics and Linguistics, pp. 157–164. London: Whurr.

Howard S, Varley R (1996) A perceptual, electropalatographic and acoustic analysis of a case of severe acquired apraxia of speech. In Powell T (ed), Pathologies of Speech and Language: Contributions of Clinical Phonetics and Linguistics, pp. 237–245. New Orleans: ICPLA.

Itoh M, Sasanuma S, Hirose H, Yoshioka, H, Ushijima T (1980) Abnormal articulatory dynamics in a patient with apraxia of speech: X-ray microbeam observation. Brain and Language, 11: 66–75.

Johnson JP, Sommers RK, Weidner WE (1977) Dichotic ear preference in aphasia. Journal of Speech Language and Hearing Research, 20: 116–29.

Johnson K (1997) Acoustic and Auditory Phonetics. Oxford: Blackwell.

Kaneko T, Uchida K, Suzuki H et al. (1981) Ultrasonic observations of vocal fold vibrations. In Stevens KN, Nirano M (eds) Vocal Fold Physiology, pp. 107–118. Tokyo: University of Tokyo Press.

Kent R (1996) Developments in the theoretical understanding of speech and its disorders. In Ball MJ, Duckworth M (eds), Advances in Clinical Phonetics pp. 1–26. Amsterdam: Benjamins.

Kent R, Read C (1992) The Acoustic Analysis of Speech. San Diego: Singular.

Kimura D (1961a) Some effects of temporal lobe damage on auditory perception. Canadian Journal of Psychology, 15: 156–165.

Kimura D (1961b) Cerebral dominance and the perception of verbal stimuli. Canadian Journal of Psychology, 15: 166–171.

Kimura D (1964) Left–right differences in the perception of melodies. Quarterly Journal of Experimental Psychology, 16: 355–58.

Ladefoged P (1967) Three Areas of Experimental Phonetics. Oxford: Oxford University Press.

Ladefoged P (1993) A Course in Phonetics, 3rd Edition. Fort Worth, Tex: Harcourt Brace.

Lakshminarayanan A, Lee S, McCutcheon M (1991) MR imaging of the vocal tract during vowel production. Journal of Magnetic Resonance Imaging, 1: 71–76.

Lass N (ed) (1996) Principles of Experimental Phonetics. St Louis: Mosby.

Laver J (1980) The Phonetic Description of Voice Quality. Cambridge: Cambridge University Press.

Laver J (1994) Principles of Phonetics. Cambridge: Cambridge University Press.

Mackay D (1968) Metamorphosis of a critical interval: age-linked changes in the delay of auditory feedback that produces maximum disruption of speech. Journal of the Acoustical Society of America, 43: 1–21.

Masaki S, Tiede M, Honda K, Shimada Y, Fujimoto I, Nakamura Y, Ninomiya N (1999) MRI-based speech production study using a synchronized sampling method. Journal of the Acoustical Society of Japan, 20: 375–379.

Milroy J (1981) Regional Accents of English: Belfast. Belfast: Blackstaff.

Moore C (1992) The correspondence of vocal tract resonance with volumes obtained from magnetic resonance images. Journal of Speeche and Hearing Research, 35: 1009–1023.

Morris P (1986) Nuclear Magnetic Resonance Imaging in Medicine and Biology. Oxford: Oxford University Press.

Narayanan S, Alwan A, Haer K (1995) An articulatory study of fricative consonants using magnetic resonance imaging. Journal of the Acoustical Society of America, 98: 1325–1347.

Orton ST (1928) A physiological theory of reading disability and stuttering in children. New England Journal of Medicine, 199: 1045–1052.

Packman A, Onslow M, Richard F, van Doorn J (1996) Syllabic stress and variability: a model of stuttering. Clinical Linguistics and Phonetics, 10: 235–262.

Peterson G, Barney H (1952) Control methods used in a study of the vowels. Journal of the Acoustical Society of America, 32: 693–703.

Perkell JS, Cohen MH, Svirsky MA et al (1992) Electromagnetic midsagittal articulometer system for transducing speech articulatory movements. Journal of the Acoustical Society of America, 92: 3078–3096.

Pettit JM, Noll JD (1979) Cerebral dominance in aphasia recovery. Brain and Language, 7: 191–200.

Prosek RA, Montgomery AA, Welden BE, Hawkins DB (1987) Formant frequencies of stuttered and fluent vowels. Journal of Speech Language and Hearing Research, 30: 301–305.

Rokkaku M, Hashimoto K, Imaizumi S, Niimi S, Kiritani S (1986) Measurements of the three-dimensional stage of the vocal tract based on the magnetic resonance imaging technique. Annual Bulletin Research Institute of Logopedics and Phoniatrics, 20: 47–54.

Ryalls J (1996) A Basic Introduction to Speech Perception. San Diego: Singular.

Ryan BP, Van Kirk B (1974) Re-establishment, transfer and maintenance of fluent speech in 50 stutterers using delayed auditory feedback and operant procedures. Journal of Speech and Hearing Disorders, 39: 3–10.

Sark S, Kalinowski J, Armson J, Stuart A (1993) Stuttering amelioration at various auditory feedback delays and speech rates. Paper presented at the annual convention of the American Speech-Language-Hearing Association, Anaheim, Calif.

Schönle PW, Wenig P, Schrader J, Hohne J, Brockmann E, Conrad B (1987) Electromagnetic articulography — use of alternating magnetic fields for tracking movements of multiple points inside and outside the vocal tract. Brain and Language, 31: 26–35.

Shprintzen RJ, Croft CB, Befkman MD, Rakoff SJ (1980) Velophryngeal insufficiency in the facio-auriculo-vertebral malformation complex. Cleft Palate Journal, 17: 132–137.

Shriberg L, Lof G (1991) Reliability studies in broad and narrow transcription. Clinical Linguistics and Phonetics, 5: 225–279.

Sparks R, Geschwind N (1968) Dichotic listening in man after section of neocortical commisures. Cortex, 4: 3–16.

Sparks R, Goodglas H, Nickel B (1970) Ipsilateral versus contralateral extinction in dichotic listening resulting from hemispheric lesions. Cortex, 6: 249–260.

Tatham MAA and Morton K(1997) Recording and displaying speech. In Ball MJ, Code C (eds), Instrumental Clinical Phonetics, pp. 1–21. London: Whurr.

Travis LE (1931) Speech Pathology. New York: Appleton-Century.

Throneburg RN, Yairi E (1994) Temporal dynamics of repetitions during the early stage of childhood stuttering: an acoustic study. Journal of Speech Language and Hearing Research, 37: 1067–1075.

Tuller B, Shao S, Kelso, JAS (1990) An evaluation of an alternating magnetic field device for monitoring tongue movements. Journal of the Acoustical Society of America, 88: 674–679.

Westbrook C, Kaut C (1993) MRI in Practice. Oxford: Blackwell.

Westbrook C (1994) Handbook of MRI Technique. Oxford: Blackwell.

Yang C-S, Kasuya H (1994) Accurate measurement of vocal tract shapes from magnetic resonance images of child, female and male subjects. Proceedings of the International Congress of Speech and Language Processing 1994, 623–626.

Yaruss JS, Conture EG (1993) F2 transitions during sound/syllable repetitions of children who stutter and predictions of stuttering chronicity. Journal of Speech Language and Hearing Research, 36: 883–896.

Zajac D, Yates C (1997) Speech aerodynamics. In Ball MJ, Code C (eds), Instrumental Clinical Phonetics, pp. 87–118. London: Whurr.

Zimmerman G (1980) Stuttering: a disorder of movement. Journal of Speech Language and Hearing Research, 23: 122–136.

Appendix

Chart 1: The International Phonetic Alphabet

THE INTERNATIONAL PHONETIC ALPHABET (revised to 1993, corrected 1996)

CONSONANTS (PULMONIC)

	Bilabial	Labiodental	Dental	Alveolar	Postalveolar	Retroflex	Palatal	Velar	Uvular	Pharyngeal	Glottal
Plosive	p b			t d		ʈ ɖ	c ɟ	k g	q ɢ		ʔ
Nasal	m	ɱ		n		ɳ	ɲ	ŋ	N		
Trill	B			r					R		
Tap or Flap				ɾ		ɽ					
Fricative	ɸ β	f v	θ ð	s z	ʃ ʒ	ʂ ʐ	ç ʝ	x ɣ	χ ʁ	ħ ʕ	h ɦ
Lateral fricative				ɬ ɮ							
Approximant		ʋ		ɹ		ɻ	j	ɰ			
Lateral approximant				l		ɭ	ʎ	L			

Where symbols appear in pairs, the one to the right represents a voiced consonant. Shaded areas denote articulations judged impossible.

CONSONANTS (NON-PULMONIC)

Clicks		Voiced implosives		Ejectives	
ʘ	Bilabial	ɓ	Bilabial	'	Examples:
ǀ	Dental	ɗ	Dental/alveolar	p'	Bilabial
ǃ	(Post)alveolar	ʄ	Palatal	t'	Dental/alveolar
ǂ	Palatoalveolar	ɠ	Velar	k'	Velar
ǁ	Alveolar lateral	ʛ	Uvular	s'	Alveolar fricative

OTHER SYMBOLS

ʍ Voiceless labial-velar fricative
w Voiced labial-velar approximant
ɥ Voiced labial-palatal approximant
H Voiceless epiglottal fricative
ʕ Voiced epiglottal fricative
ʡ Epiglottal plosive

ɕ ʑ Alveolo-palatal fricatives
ɺ Alveolar lateral flap
ɧ Simultaneous ʃ and x

Affricates and double articulations can be represented by two symbols joined by a tie bar if necessary.

k͡p t͡s

VOWELS

Where symbols appear in pairs, the one to the right represents a rounded vowel.

SUPRASEGMENTALS

'	Primary stress	ˌfoʊnəˈtɪʃən
ˌ	Secondary stress	
ː	Long	eː
ˑ	Half-long	eˑ
˘	Extra-short	ĕ
ǀ	Minor (foot) group	
ǁ	Major (intonation) group	
.	Syllable break	ɹi.ækt
‿	Linking (absence of a break)	

DIACRITICS Diacritics may be placed above a symbol with a descender, e.g. ŋ̊

Voiceless	n̥ d̥	Breathy voiced	b̤ a̤	Dental	t̪ d̪
Voiced	s̬ t̬	Creaky voiced	b̰ a̰	Apical	t̺ d̺
Aspirated	tʰ dʰ	Linguolabial	t̼ d̼	Laminal	t̻ d̻
More rounded	ɔ̹	Labialized	tʷ dʷ	Nasalized	ẽ
Less rounded	ɔ̜	Palatalized	tʲ dʲ	Nasal release	dⁿ
Advanced	u̟	Velarized	tˠ dˠ	Lateral release	dˡ
Retracted	e̠	Pharyngealized	tˤ dˤ	No audible release	d̚
Centralized	ë	Velarized or pharyngealized	ɫ		
Mid-centralized	ě	Raised	e̝	(ɹ̝ = voiced alveolar fricative)	
Syllabic	n̩	Lowered	e̞	(β̞ = voiced bilabial approximant)	
Non-syllabic	e̯	Advanced Tongue Root	e̘		
Rhoticity	ɚ a˞	Retracted Tongue Root	e̙		

TONES AND WORD ACCENTS

LEVEL			CONTOUR		
e̋ or	˥ Extra high	ě or	˩˥ Rising
é	˦ High	ê	˥˩ Falling
ē	˧ Mid	e᷄	˦˥ High rising
è	˨ Low	e᷅	˩˨ Low rising
ȅ	˩ Extra low	e᷈	˧˦˨ Rising-falling
↓	Downstep	↗	Global rise
↑	Upstep	↘	Global fall

127

Chart 2: The Extensions to the International Phonetic Alphabet

extIPA SYMBOLS FOR DISORDERED SPEECH
(Revised to 1997)

CONSONANTS (other than those on the IPA Chart)

	bilabial	labiodental	dentolabial	labioalv.	linguolabial	interdental	bidental	alveolar	velar	velophar.
Plosive			p̪ b̪	p̺ b̺	t̼ d̼	t̪ d̪				
Nasal			m̪	m̺	n̼	n̪				
Trill					r̼	r̪				
Fricative median			f̪ v̪	f̺ v̺	θ̼ ð̼	θ̪ ð̪	ɦ̪ ɦ̪			fŋ
Fricative lateral+median								ʪ ʫ		
Fricative nareal	m̃							ñ̰	ŋ̰̃	
Percussive	w̰ w̰						ʭ			
Approximant lateral					l̼	l̪				

DIACRITICS

↔ labial spreading	s̳	‖ strong articulation	f̬	~ denasal	m̃
˷ dentolabial	v̪	˒ weak articulation	v̬	˙~ nasal escape	ṽ̰
˗ interdental/bidental	n̰	\ reiterated articulation	p\p\p	≈ velopharyngeal friction	s̰̃
= alveolar	t̠	˔ whistled articulation	s̝	↓ ingressive airflow	p↓
˷ linguolabial	d̼	→ sliding articulation	θs	↑ egressive airflow	!↑

CONNECTED SPEECH

(.) short pause
(..) medium pause
(...) long pause
f loud speech [{*f* laʊd *f*}]
ff louder speech [{*ff* laʊdɚ *ff*}]
p quiet speech [{*p* kwaɪət *p*}]
pp quieter speech [{*pp* kwaɪətə *pp*}]
allegro fast speech [{*allegro* fɑːst *allegro*}]
lento slow speech [{ *lento* sloʊ *lento*}]
crescendo, ralentando, etc may also be used

VOICING

pre-voicing	ˌz
post-voicing	z̦
partial devoicing	(z̦)
initial partial devoicing	(z̦
final partial devoicing	z̦)
partial voicing	(s̬)
initial partial voicing	(s̬
final partial voicing	s̬)
= unaspirated	p=
ʰ pre-aspiration	ʰp

OTHERS

(̄) indeterminate sound	(( )) extraneous noise ((2 sylls))
(V̄), (Pl) indeterminate vowel, plosive, etc	¡ sublaminal lower alveolar percussive click
(Pl,vls) indeterminate voiceless plosive, etc	!¡ alveolar & sublaminal click ('cluck-click')
( ) silent articulation (ʃ), (m)	* sound with no available symbol

Chart 3: The VoQS Voice Quality Symbols

VoQS: Voice Quality Symbols

AIRSTREAM TYPES

Œ	oesophageal speech	Ɯ	electrolarynx speech
IO	tracheo-oesophageal speech	↓	pulmonic ingressive speech

PHONATION TYPES

V	modal voice	F	falsetto
W	whisper	C	creak
V̤	whispery voice (murmur)	V̰	creaky voice
Ç	whispery creak	V!	harsh voice
V!!	ventricular phonation	V̰!!	diplophonia
V̩	anterior or pressed phonation	W̲	posterior whisper

SUPRALARYNGEAL SETTINGS

L̝	raised larynx	L̞	lowered larynx
V�œ	labialized voice (open round)	Vʷ	labialized voice (close round)
V↔	spread-lip voice	Vᶹ	labio-dentalized voice
V̺	linguo-apicalized voice	V̻	linguo-laminalized voice
V˞	retroflex voice	V̪	dentalized voice
V̲	alveolarized voice	V̲ʲ	palatoalveolarized voice
Vʲ	palatalized voice	Vˠ	velarized voice
Vʁ	uvularized voice	Vˤ	pharyngealized voice
V̰ˤ	laryngo-pharyngealized voice	Vᴴ	faucalized voice
Ṽ	nasalized voice	V̄	denasalized voice
J̞	open jaw voice	J̝	close jaw voice
J̰	right offset jaw voice	J̧	left offset jaw voice
J̰	protruded jaw voice	Θ	protruded tongue voice

USE OF LABELED BRACES & NUMERALS TO MARK STRETCHES OF
SPEECH AND DEGREES AND COMBINATIONS OF VOICE QUALITY

['ðɪs ɪz 'nɔ·məl 'vɔɪs {3V! 'ðɪs ɪz 'veɹi 'hɑ·ʃ 'vɔɪs 3V!} 'ðɪs ɪz 'nɔ·məl 'vɔɪs
wʌns 'mɔ˞ {L̝1V! 'ðɪs ɪz 'les 'hɑ·ʃ 'vɔɪs wɪð 'loʊəd 'læɹɪŋks 1V!L̝}]

Index

Aberdeen Speech Aid, 96
  see also auditory feedback, delayed
accent, regional transcription of, 19
  see also diacritics
acoustic analysis, 65–7
  of segment duration, 84–7
acoustic instrumentation, chapter 6
    passim
acoustic measurement, 67–72
acoustic phonetics, 61
acoustic transmission theory, 56
acoustic waveform, 115
acquired articulation disorder, 49
acquired language disorder, *see* aphasia
acquired neurological disorders, 6
additions, 6
  and delayed auditory feedback, 100
aerometry, 42, 58
affricates
  acoustic characteristics of, 69
  transcription of, 19
air pressure, intra-oral, and cleft palate, 4
airflow; airstream
  egressive, 42, 58
  ingressive, 6, 58, 74
  measurement of, 44
  nasal, 42, 43–4, 58
  oral, 42
alveolar
  –postalveolar contact pattern, 50
  realized as palatovelar, 53
  targets, 38, 53
  –velar contrast, 38, 53

Americanist tradition, 10
  see also International Phonetic
    Alphabet
aphasia, 6–7, 101–2
  Broca's type, 6, 84–7
  conduction, 101
  and delayed auditory feedback, 96
  and left-ear advantage/preference,
    97–8
  Wernicke's type, 6, 107–8
approximants, 4, 38
apraxia, 7, 49
  and delayed auditory feedback, 96
  and vowel duration, 68, 86
  and X-ray microbeam analysis, 48
articulation
  alveolar, 15
  bidental, 27
  bilabial, 15
  dentolabial, 27
  and electropalatography, 44–5
  imaging techniques, 45–8
  interdental, 27
  labio-alveolar, 27
  labio-dental, 15
  place of, 15, 27, 44
  reiterated 29
  silent, 31
  sliding, 29
  transcription errors, 50
  velar, 15
  velopharyngeal, 27

articulatory instrumentation, chapter 4
    passim
artificial palate, *see* electropalatography
artificial stutter, 100–1
audiograms, 90, 91
audiometry, 90–1
    pure tone, 90–1
    speech, 91
audiotapes, transcription of, 21
auditory feedback, 91–3
    delayed, 95–6, 99–103
    gamma-loop, 92, 93
    instrumentation, 96
    kinaesthetic, 92, 93
    and speech production, 8
    and stutter, 96
    tactile, 92, 93
auditory recognition system, *see* cardinal
    vowel system
auditory system, 88–9

bark scale, 94
brain lesion, and auditory pathway,
    105–8
    see also acquired neurological
        disorders; hearing
breathy voice, 6
    see also voice quality

cardinal vowel system, 18, 21
clicks, 16–17
    see also consonants, non-pulmonic
child speech disorders, 5; *see also* devel-
    opmental articulation disorder
cleft palate, 3–4, 50–3
    and electropalatography, 49
    and hypernasality, 58
    and place contrasts, 38
    X-ray analysis of, 46
cluttering, 5, 6
cognitive phonetics, 117, 118
comprehension, 88
computerization
    and delayed auditory feedback, 96
    imaging of air flow, 42
    of transcription, 22
    of vocal fold activity, 43
connected speech, 71

and magnetic resonance imaging
    studies, 57
transcription of, 29, 30
consonants, 11
    IPA chart, 15
    labial, 8, 52
    non-pulmonic, 16
    obstruent, 7
    sonorant, 7
    voiced/voiceless, 4, 15
contrastivity, and cleft palate, 38
covert contrasts, 53, 54
craniofacial disorders, 3–4
    X-ray analysis of, 46
    see also cleft palate; Pierre Robin
        sequence
creaky voice, 5, 6, 71–2
    see also voice quality

deafness
    central, 90
    conductive, 89–90
    pre- and postlingual, 8
    sensorineural, 90
    see also ear, structure of; hearing
developmental articulation disorder, 49
diacritics, 20–1, 30–1
    to denote regional accent, 19
    and disordered speech, 21
    and extIPA chart, 29
dichotic listening, 96–8, 99, 104–8
diphthongs, 19
    acoustic characteristics of, 68–9
    diphthongization, 8
disfluency, 5–6, 49. 100–1
disordered speech, chapter 3 passim
    acoustic analysis, 73
    articulatory analysis, chapter 5 passim
    auditory analysis, chapter 9 passim
    perceptual analysis, chapter 9 passim
double articulation, 19, 51, 52
dysarthria, 7, 39–40, 49
    and delayed auditory feedback, 96
dysprosody, 6

ear, structure of, 88–9; *see also* deafness;
    hearing impairment; right-ear
    advantage

ejectives, 16–17
 see also consonants, non-pulmonic
electroglottograph, 43
electrolaryngography, 43, 70–1, 111–12, 113
electromagnetic articulography, 48, 111, 114, 116
electromyography, 41–2, 111. 116
electropalatography, 44, 49–55, 111, 112, 114
 and cleft palate (case study), 50–2
 feedback, 52
 with nasal airflow and acoustic waveform, 115
 and stroke (case study), 49–50
endoscopy, 43
extIPA symbols, 26–32, 128

feedback
 auditory, 91–3
 delayed, 95–6, 99–103
 gamma-loop, 92, 93
 kinaesthetic, 92, 93
 tactile, 92, 93
formants, 65, 67
 frequency, 65, 67, 84
 structure and intelligibility, 67
frequency, 63–4, 94
 see also fundamental frequency
fricatives, 15, 16, 27–8, 84–5
 acoustic characteristics of, 69
 alveolar, 51
 bidental, 28
 dental, 27
 duration, 84, 86
 fortis, 85, 86
 glottal, 28
 interdental, 27
 lenis, 85, 86
 magnetic resonance imaging studies, 57
 nasalized, 4
 palato-alveolar, 50, 51, 52
 velopharyngeal, 6, 75
 voiced/voiceless, 7, 63
 voiceless waveform, 63
 whistled, 29
fronting, 37

fundamental frequency, 63, 64, 67, 93
 and delayed auditory feedback, 95
Fx waveform, 71

glottal stop, 16
 substitute for non-labial consonant, 8

harmonics, 64, 67
head injury
 and acquired neurological disorder, 6
 and dichotic listening, 104–7
hearing, 88
 extinction patterns, 105, 106–7
 impairment, 8
 loss, 89–90
 see also audiometry; auditory feedback; deafness; dichotic listening; ear, structure of; left-ear advantage/preference; right-ear advantage hemispheric dominance/specialization, 97, 104
 retraining, 107–8
hesitation noises, 12
hypernasality, 4
 and cleft palate, 58, 59
hyponasality, and hearing impairment, 58, 59

imaging techniques, 44, 45–8
implosives, 16–17
 see also consonants, non-pulmonic
initiation of speech, 42
insertion, and delayed auditory feedback, 100
instrumentation, 2, 21–2
 auditory and perceptual, chapter 8 passim
 combined techniques, 111–14
 investigations of disordered speech, chapter 5 passim
intelligibility, 4
intensity, 64
International Phonetic Alphabet, 10, 14–21, 127
 accent, 16
 cardinal vowels, 18, 20
 consonant chart, 15–16
 diacritics, 20–1

non-pulmonic chart, 16–17
suprasegmentals, 17
vowels chart, 17–18, 19
see also extIPA; transcription
intonation, 1, 4, 6, 8, 11, 70, 71

Kent Model of Speech Organization and
    Disorders, 117, 118

laryngoscopy, 111
larynx, laryngeal activity, 4, 42, 43, 111
left-ear advantage/preference, 97
    see also dichotic listening;
        hemispheric dominance/specializa-
        tion
linear predictive coding, 81–3
lip shape
    harmonization, 37–8
    rounding, 67
liquids, acoustic characteristics, 69–70
lisp, 37
loudness, 1, 11, 94
    and delayed auditory feedback, 95
    and hearing impairment, 8
    and stutter, 6
    transcription of, 30
    Lx waveform, 112

magnetic resonance imaging, 47, 55–8
    data errors, 56–7
mel scale, 93
mispronunciation and delayed auditory
    feedback, 95
monophthongization, 8
mouthing, 31
muscle activity of speech, 41–2

nasal resonance, 43, 59
nasal snort, *see* velopharyngeal
    fricative/snort
nasal stop, 15, 43–4
    substituted for plosive stop, 4
nasality, 4, 32, 58
nasals, 50, 51
    acoustic characteristics of, 70
    magnetic resonance imaging studies,
        57
NasalView, 58, 59

nasometry, 44, 58–60
neurophonetics, 3
nuclear magnetic resonance, 56

omissions, and delayed auditory
    feedback, 95, 100
oral/nasal sound contast, 3–4, 39
orthography, English, 12–13

paraphrasia
    phonemic, 102
    phonological, 6
    semantic, 6
Parkinsonism
    and delayed auditory feedback, 96,
        102–3
    X-ray microbeam diagnosis, 48
pauses
    filled/unfilled, 6
    transcription of, 12, 29
perception, 88
percussives, 28
periodic sound, 62, 63–4
perseveration, 6
phon scale, 94
phonation, 42–3
phonemic substitution, 37
phonetics
    acoustic, 2
    articulatory, 2, 3
    auditory, 3
    definition, 1
    perceptual, 3
    phonetic realization, 5
Phonic Mirror, 96
    see also auditory feedback, delayed
phonology, 10
    phonological contrast, 34
    phonological organization, 5
    phonological neutralization, 81
PhonX, 96
    see also auditory feedback, delayed
Pierre Robin sequence, 49, 52–3
pitch, 4, 64, 70, 93, 94, 111–12
    see also intonation; mel scale
place contrast
    and cleft palate, 38
    and Pierre Robin sequence, 52

plosives, 4, 16, 28
  acoustic characteristics, 69
  alveolar, 50, 51, 52
  labiodental, 8
  voiced, voiceless, 28, 34–5
  word-initial, 34
prosody, 11
  and stutter, 117
PSL (portable speech laboratory), 59–60
psychoacoustics, 93–5
  measurement, 93–4
pulmonic egressive speech transcription, 42
pulmonic ingressive speech transcription, 29, 42

radiography, 45–6
reiteration, 75, 76, 78, 79
repetition, 6, 75
  and delayed auditory feedback, 95, 100
resonance, 64–5
rhythm, 1, 11
right-ear advantage, 97
  see also hemispheric dominance/specialization

segment duration, 84–7
segmental duration, 67, 68
sine wave, 62
sone scale, 94
sound spectrum, 65, 66
sound waves, 61–3
spectograms, 66–7, 76–8, 82–3, 86
spectograph, 65–6, 67
speech
  acoustics, 61
  audiometry, 91
  production, 2; errors, 102
  segments, 11
  sounds, 1; extralinguistic, 1
spring mass, 64, 65
stops
  glottal, 8, 16
  nasal, 4, 15, 43–4
  nasalized, 4
  plosive, 4, 15

stress, 11
  and hearing impairment, 8
  syllabic, 118–19
stroke/acquired neurological disorder, 6
  and speech error (case study), 49
structural imaging, see magnetic resonance imaging; radiography; ultrasound
stuttering, 5, 101
  case study, 73–5
  and delayed auditory feedback, 96
  model, 117, 118–19
  and voice onset time, 68
subphonemic cues, 53
substitutions, 6
  and delayed auditory feedback, 95, 100
suprasegmentals, 5, 6, 11, 17
symbolization, 2
  of disordered speech, 25–32
  of voice quality, 32
  see also accent; diacritics; extIPA; International Phonetic Alphabet
symbol systems, 10
  phonetic, 13
  see also extIPA; International Phonetic Alphabet

tempo, 1, 11
  and cluttering/stuttering, 6
  and delayed auditory feedback, 95
  and hearing impairment, 8
  transcription of, 30
tongue
  movement and ultrasound, 46
  –palate placement, 44, 49, 50, 51, 53, 58
  pattern, 45
tracking, see electromagnetic articulography; X-ray microbeam
transcription, chapter 2 passim
  broad, 22–3, 34–5
  computerization of, 22
  of disordered speech, chapter 3 passim
  impressionistic, 2, 10, 50, 114–19
  instrumental, 2

live, 21
narrow, 22, 23, 34–5
of recorded data, 21
reliability, 22, 36, 116–17
see also extIPA; International Phonetic
   Alphabet
transposition, 6

ultrasound, 46
see also imaging techniques

variability, and stuttering, 117
velar substitution, 50, 51
velic action, 43–4
velopharyngeal inadequacy, *see* craniofacial disorders
velopharyngeal fricative/snort, 28, 75
ventricular folds, substituted for vocal
   folds, 5
videotape recordings, transcription from,
   21
Visi-Pitch, 71
vocal fold
   activity, 42–3, 111
   disorders of, 4
   vibration, vibration frequency, 43, 64
vocal tract, 65
   measurement, modelling, 56, 57
voice
   modal, 71
   palatalized, 72
   supraglottal, 72
   velarized, 72
voice disorder
   and intelligibility, 4
   and voice quality, 5

voice onset time, 67
   and stuttering, 68
voice quality, 5, 6, 11, 71–2
   symbolization of, 32–4
   see also breathy voice; creaky voice
voicing, 29
   errors, 100
VoQS system, 32, 33, 129
vowels
   acoustic characteristics of, 68
   central, 19
   centralization, 67
   closed, 68
   diphthongs, 19
   disordered, 19, 80–4
   duration, 67–8, 86, 117
   formant frequency, 84
   formant structure, 68, 84
   lax, 19, 68
   neutralization, 81
   open, 68
   production, 56
   rounded, 81
   tense, 68
   transcription of, 19, 21, 80
   waveform, 63
   see also cardinal vowel system

whisper, 71, 72
word-finding difficulty, 6
word-initial
   plosives, 34
   sound blocking, 74

X-ray, 45–6
X-ray microbeam, 47–8
   see also imaging techniques